LONG-TERM CARE CASE MANAGEMENT: DESIGN AND EVALUATION

Robert A. Applebaum, Ph.D., is an associate professor in the department of sociology and a research fellow at the Scripps Gerontology Center at Miami University in Oxford, Ohio. He has been involved in the evaluation of case management programs since 1978, including work on the Wisconsin Community Care Organization, Wisconsin Community Options Program, Ohio's PASSPORT program, and the National Long-Term Care Channeling Demonstration.

Dr. Applebaum has served the Gerontological Society of America (GSA) as a member of GSA's public policy committee, as a book review editor for *The Gerontologist*, and has spoken frequently at national and state conferences on home care. Author of numerous articles, monographs, and a book on community-based long-term care, Dr. Applebaum served as a guest editor of a special issue on quality assurance published by the American Society on Aging in its journal, *Generations*. Dr. Applebaum received a Ph.D. from the University of Wisconsin-Madison; a M.S.W. from Ohio State University, and a B.A. from Ohio University.

Carol D. Austin, Ph.D., is an associate professor at the College of Social Work, Ohio State University and is currently a member of the Commission on Families of the National Association of Social Work. She chaired the social research, planning and practice section of the Gerontological Society of America between 1986–1988. From 1988–1990 she served as the director of the Ohio Department of Aging and was involved in securing passage of Ohio's Eldercare Initiative.

Since 1975 Dr. Austin has been involved in long-term care with a focus on the role of case management in the delivery of community-based services. She has worked on the Wisconsin Community Care Organization, the Social/HMO, private long-term care insurance at Group Health Corporation of Puget Sound, a four-state comparative study of case management in community-based long-term care in the Pacific Northwest, and with the Veterans Administration Health Services Research & Development program. Dr. Austin is a frequent speaker at national conferences and has authored numerous articles and books. She is a member of the editorial boards of the journals *Health and Social Work*, and *Generations*. Dr. Austin received a Ph.D. from the University of Wisconsin-Madison; a M.S.W. from the University of Michigan; and a B.A. from the City College of New York.

Long-Term Care Case Management:
Design and Evaluation

Robert Applebaum, Ph.D., M.S.W.

Carol Austin, Ph.D., M.S.W.

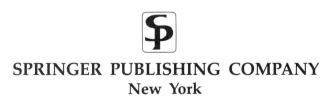

SPRINGER PUBLISHING COMPANY
New York

Springer Publishing Company, Inc.
536 Broadway
New York, NY 10012

90 91 92 93 94 / 5 4 3 2 1

Applebaum, Robert.
    Long-term care case management : design and evaluation / Robert Applebaum, Carol Austin.
        p.   cm.
    Includes bibliographical references.
    ISBN 0-8261-6430-7
    1. Long-term care of the sick.   2. Long-term care facilities.
I. Austin, Carol D.   II. Title.
    [DNLM: 1. Long Term Care.   2. Patient Care Planning.   3. Quality Assurance, Health Care—United States.   WX 162 A648L]
RA564.8.A65   1990
362.1'6—dc20
DNLM/DLC
for Library of Congress   90-9483
                                                                   CIP

Printed in the United States of America

Contents

PART III.   PAST EXPERIENCES AND FUTURE CHALLENGES

Preface

Several years ago at a national conference we were presenting a session on a new "hot" topic called case management. To introduce the presentation we had asked a colleague (Dr. James Callahan) to say a few words about case management. Much to our surprise, rather than talking about the rise in case management, the speaker pulled out a newspaper and began to read the following:

> Reuters News Service—Dateline Cairo, Egypt
>
> Archaeologists today uncovered the remains of a person whom they believe to be history's first case manager. Archaeologists believe that the woman became lost in a sandstorm on her way home from meeting a group of nomad providers. They speculate that she was trying to convince the providers to use her comprehensive assessment. Archaeologists theorize that she was crushed to death under the weight of her hieroglyphic assessment tablets.

Although the facts may be disputed, this fictitious story makes the point that some form of case management has been a part of the health and human service system for a very long time. What is less clear, however, is what case-managed care actually is and what its role should be in the long-term care delivery system. To this end, the purpose of this volume is to provide readers with a broadly based synthesis of information regarding case management program design and evaluation.

The authors have been privileged to have been involved with a wide range of long-term care programs that include case management services. Case management has become omnipresent, even when there is limited consensus about just what it is. In some quarters case management may be considered a fad, while elsewhere it is viewed as a panacea. In either event, experience illustrates that virtually every provider claims to provide case management service, and this is the case even when there is little consensus about what it is and even when there is limited evidence to demonstrate its effectiveness. Case management remains a frequently controversial cornerstone in the provision of community-based long-term care services.

This volume brings together two essential aspects of case management: design and evaluation. The book is organized into three parts. Chapters 1 through 4 are primarily focused on design issues; Chapters 5 through 7 examine evaluative considerations; and the final two chapters document past experiences and future challenges.

Chapter 1 provides an overview of the case management landscape, addressing definitional and contextual variables. Three basic models of case management are introduced in this chapter: broker, service management, and managed care. Causes of the apparent widespread popularity of case management service provision are identified and discussed. The core components of case management are examined in Chapter 2. This chapter draws heavily on the experience of various long-term care demonstration projects to illustrate how the components of case management were implemented with considerable variation among the projects.

Far too often, analyses of case management have failed to take into consideration the impact of the program within which case management services are delivered. In order to understand that programmatic constraints limit how case managers can perform, it is necessary to thoroughly examine the programmatic context case managers face. Chapter 3 introduces four critical program variables which, taken together, shape the character of the case management service. These programmatic variables are: financing/reimbursement, targeting criteria, gatekeeping, and organizational auspices. Cross program/project comparisons are made for each programmatic variable, demonstrating how any specific case management service can vary on a number of dimensions. Chapter 4 focuses attention on a number of major design options that require attention in the design of case management services. These options include: local delivery system impact, tasks and functions, staffing, level of professionalization, authority, interface with the health care system, timing of case management intervention, caseload size, case mix, and service intensity.

Although there has been considerable demonstration and programmatic experience with the provision of case management services, relatively little information about how to demonstrate the effectiveness of the service has been produced. Chapter 5 emphasizes the need to distinguish among three critical concepts: quality, evaluation, and quality assurance. Three evaluative approaches (descriptive measures, program review, and program impact) and three quality assurance methods (structural, process, and outcomes) are introduced and analyzed. Chapters 6 and 7 respectively examine quality assurance and impact evaluation in greater depth.

Case management service design and implementation have evolved over time. Chapter 8 presents an evolutionary view of this development, noting the apparent movement away from reliance on the broker model toward case management approaches which incorporate more direct financial authority and accountability for the case manager. This retrospective, longitudinal analysis illustrates how case management program design and practice have shifted in response to a changing policy environment (1971–1986).

Agencies considering the development of case management services must confront several significant planning issues. Chapter 9 specifies these critical diagnostic questions and examines implications of various responses. Case management is provided in an extremely complex service delivery environment. Program developers, practitioners, and administrators must be equipped with sharp diagnostic skills, a firm conceptual foundation, and a well honed set of management indicators. These are the fundamentals. These are the basic tools for long-term care case management design and evaluation.

ROBERT APPLEBAUM
CAROL AUSTIN

Acknowledgments

In a very real sense, this volume has its origins in the early days of its authors' professional development. We are members of that cohort of researchers whose careers grew along with the development of community-based long-term care demonstration projects. This interdisciplinary cadre of analysts focused its efforts and energies on the development of community-based long-term care delivery systems, their design, financing, organization, service delivery experience, and effects. This volume represents over 25 years of the authors' experience with the care and feeding of programmatic intitiatives aimed at helping elders remain in their own homes and communities.

Early drafts of the design chapters of this book were developed under a grant from the Administration on Aging to the University of Washington, Institute on Aging, to operate the Pacific Northwest Long Term Care Gerontology Center. This volume would not have been possible without the assistance of a number of colleagues at the University of Washington. Jan Lowe assisted with gathering literature and primary source documents. Kathleen O'Connor's editorial skills contributed to the readability of early drafts. Dorothy Sjaastad provided much valued clerical support. Ed Borgatta, then Director of the Center, provided methodological direction and moral support.

The section on evaluation and quality assurance of case management has been shaped by work on several major evaluation studies, including the Wisconsin Community Care Project and the National Channeling Demonstration. In particular, Peter Kemper, the lead investigator on the channeling project, influenced the nature of this section. Support from the Fred Meyer Charitable Trust provided assistance to this effort as well.

At the Scripps Gerontology Center at Miami University, several people have contributed to this effort. Darlene Davidson and Thelma Carmack prepared the manuscript. Mary Sohngen provided her expert editing and organizational skills to the work. Finally, our colleagues at Scripps provided an environment that stimulated and encouraged this work.

Part I

DESIGNING CASE MANAGEMENT

Our plans miscarry because they have no aim. When a man does not know what harbor he is making for, no wind is the right wind. SENECA (4 B.C.–A.D. 65)

Nothing is more terrible than activity without insight. CARLYLE (1795–1881)

My life has no purpose, no direction, no aim, no meaning, and yet I'm happy. I can't figure out what I am doing right. CHARLES M. SCHULZ

Chapter **1**

Basic Concepts

THE EXPANSION OF COMMUNITY-BASED CARE

Although providing care to individuals in their own homes is not a new idea—provisions for in-home care were included in the first formal social welfare legislation in England in 1601—it has received renewed attention in recent years from policymakers, advocates for the elderly and disabled, and researchers. The expansion of community-based long-term care has intensified in response to the increasing elderly population, the rapidly rising cost of nursing home care, and in response to desires of older persons to remain in the community rather than being placed in nursing homes.

Concern about the institutional funding bias of the long-term care system has generated questions about the cost and appropriateness of the level of care provided to many impaired elders. Since the early 1970s there has been growing concern over the rising cost of nursing home care. The cost issue becomes even more pressing when one realizes that for every elder residing in an institutional setting, there are three others with chronic levels of functional disability living in the community (Weissert, 1985b). In an attempt to respond to increasing costs, community-based long-term care services have been advanced as a potentially cost effective way to provide care for impaired elders in their own homes, thereby obviating the need for institutional placement. The extent to which the community-based and institutional populations are alike remains a point of some contention. What is not in dispute is that institutional care is fundamentally different from community-based long-term care services in at least one area. A nursing home is a single provider with an easily accessible resident population, while the community long-term care delivery system consists of a multiplicity of providers, most of whom deliver care in the clients' homes (Seidl, Austin, & Greene, 1977).

Expansion of community-based care is primarily fueled by two major trends. First, there has been an increase in the funding that can be used for in-home and community-based services, stemming from the expansion of existing federal funding sources, such as Medicare, Medicaid, Title III of the Older Americans Act, Social Services Block grants, and volunteer programs under Action. These increases have either occurred through an expansion of benefits, e.g., Medicare, Medicaid, or a reordered set of service priorities. These factors have resulted in a dramatic increase in funding for community-based care; for example, home health products and services were estimated to cost over 9 billion dollars in 1985 (Sabatino, 1989).

The second major trend in system expansion has been the use of case coordinators, or case managers, who have responsibility for arranging and monitoring long-term care services for program clients.

Fragmentation in the provision of long-term care services has been well documented. The need to coordinate services at community, program, and client levels is of major concern. The combined need for coordination and cost containment will be present for the foreseeable future. Case management is one response to these continuing pressures. Thus, case management is widely accepted as a core component of community-based and, in some locations, institutional long-term care. Why has case management enjoyed such widespread acceptance? First, fragmented and complex delivery systems present formidable obstacles for functionally disabled persons. Second, impaired elders require assistance from multiple providers. Third, and perhaps most important, case management can generally be inserted into a community's delivery system without restructuring relationships among the providers in that system. One of the virtues of case management as a policy reform in long-term care is precisely that it can be placed within the ongoing delivery system and does not require restructuring of interorganizational relationships.

Case management has been tested in a series of over 15 federally sponsored demonstrations between 1973 and 1985 (Haskins, Capitman, Collignon, DeGraaf, Yorde, 1985; Kemper, Applebaum, & Harrigan, 1987). Federal waivers under the Medicaid Program, Section 2176, of the Omnibus Reconciliation Act of 1981, permit reimbursement for case management in waiver-funded programs operating in over 40 states. Statewide case-managed in-home long-term care programs have also been expanded. Over one-half of all states currently operate statewide case management programs. Case management is also a key ingredient in recent demonstration projects in managed health care, such as the Social/Health Maintenance Organization, the Medicare H.M.O. Projects, the Robert Wood Johnson Hospital Initatives in Long-Term Care, and in some newly developed private long-term care insurance policies. These recent developments suggest that the role and presence of long-term case management will continue to expand in a variety of delivery systems supported by different sources of funding. This chapter will introduce basic case management concepts with specific attention to goals, context, program variations, and models.

WHAT IS LONG-TERM CARE CASE MANAGEMENT?

Long-term care case management is an intervention using a human service professional (typically a nurse or social worker) to arrange and monitor an optimum package of long-term care services. Case management is certainly not a new concept. It is a service designed to coordinate multiple services provided to an individual client. Virtually all providers of direct services report managing their cases (Dronska, 1983). Thus, there are many individuals who claim to provide some type of case management in the existing system. There is, however, an important distinction to be made between the type of case management that is provided in conjunction with direct services, and comprehensive long-term care case management (Kemper, et al., 1986). Three key features distinguish comprehensive long-term care case management:

- intensity
- breadth of services encompassed, and
- duration of case management.

Intensity refers to the amount of time case managers spend with their clients. Indicators of intensity include the amount of time case managers have for providing information and support to clients and their caregivers. Caseload size is a key indicator of intensity. A case manager serving a caseload of 50 to 75 for example, can provide more intense monitoring of clients' conditions and service provision than a case manager with a caseload of 300. Practitioners providing comprehensive long-term care case management have caseload sizes that permit intense involvement with clients.

Breadth of services refers to how broadly case managers view the problems of clients. The breadth of services case managers can provide is a function of program financing, structured and comprehensive assessment, the care planning process, and supervisory review. Some agencies, for instance, have a narrow view of case management practice and may limit the services case managers arrange to include only those that can be provided by their own organization. Comprehensive long-term care case management involves a broad span of services to meet client needs.

Duration refers to how long case managers remain involved with clients. Where funding for case management is tied to a specific service (e.g., certified home health care), case management may be withdrawn when the service is no longer reimbursable despite client need. Indicators of longer term involvement between the case manager and client include formalized, scheduled reassessments and regular, systematic monitoring of a client's condition and care plan. Frail clients often require case management for extended periods. Duration of case managers' involvement is partly a function of the client's functional capacity.

These three characteristics (intensity, breadth, and duration) distinguish long-term care case management from other types of case management such as that provided by hospital discharge planners, home health agencies, and county social service departments. These agencies generally provide case management that is limited in one or more of these key features. This more clearly defined type of long-term case management has not been practiced by a majority of service providers. There has, however, been a substantial increase in long-term care case management as defined above, in many local delivery systems (Austin, Roberts, & Low, 1985).

CASE MANAGEMENT GOALS

Although there is considerable consensus on the core activities that constitute case management, there appear to be multiple goals or expectations concerning these activities. The discussion that follows begins with those goals that are primarily client-oriented and proceeds to those goals that are more far-reaching in their potential impact on the character of long-term care delivery systems. These goals are summarized in Table 1-1.

Goals That Are Primarily Client Oriented

1. To Assure That Services Given Are Appropriate to the Needs of a Particular Client. Each of the component activities of case management supports the goal of assuring that prescribed services are tai-

TABLE 1–1 Goals Associated with Case Management

Client Oriented Goals

1. To assure that services given are appropriate to the needs of a particular client.
2. To monitor the client's condition in order to guarantee the appropriateness of service.
3. To improve client access to the continuum of long-term care services.
4. To support the client's caregivers.
5. To serve as bridges between institutional and community-based care systems.

System Oriented Goals

1. To facilitate the development of a broader array of noninstitutional services.
2. To promote quality and efficiency in the delivery of long-term care services.
3. To enhance the coordination of long-term care service delivery.
4. To target individuals most at risk of nursing home placement in order to prevent inappropriate institutionalization.
5. To contain costs by controlling client access to services, especially high cost services.

lored to meet an individual client's needs. For example, assessment is comprehensive and designed to identify a client's strengths as well as weaknesses through systematic evaluation of the client's total needs. Client problems are typically interdependent and can best be addressed using a comprehensive and holistic method. By contrast, assessments by direct service providers may not be as comprehensive since their focus may only be on the portion of client needs that they can serve. The case manager organizes both formal and informal services designed to fit clients' individual situations in the care planning process. There is no standardized formula for care plans. Theoretically, since care plans represent individualized treatment protocols, no two care plans should be exactly alike. Furthermore, care plans are not static; rather, they change with regular reassessments or when the client's situation or needs change.

2. To Monitor Clients to Ensure the Appropriateness of Long-Term Care Services. Case managers monitor clients to ensure that services have begun and are satisfactory. The monitoring function facilitates quick response to temporary or permanent changes in the client's condition. Monitoring also serves a preventive function, addressing problems before they snowball and cause new problems or aggravate existing conditions.

3. To Improve Client Access to the Continuum of Long-Term Care Services. A long-term care delivery system can be a complex maze for a client seeking appropriate services. Multiple providers, differing agency regulations, and waiting lists are just a few of the hurdles elders face when attempting to obtain services. The clients who are most disabled or functionally impaired and in greatest need of services have the most difficulty dealing with the red tape involved.

Case management is designed to simplify access to services. The case manager can serve as the single point of entry and primary contact for clients. The case manager not only knows what resources are available in a local delivery system, but is also familiar with various agency eligibility requirements. The case manager becomes the channel through which the client gains access to the continuum of long-term care services in a community. This channeling function eliminates barriers between providers and creates a delivery system that is more responsive to clients' total needs.

4. To Support the Client's Caregivers. Case managers also assess and monitor the status of the clients' informal support systems. In some instances, clients have no active informal support systems, but case managers may be able to identify individuals who could provide some assistance. Caregivers often become exhausted from the demands of their responsibilities. A case manager can monitor the situation and provide additional services or respite when the informal support system is at a breaking point. This intervention can be crucial, for without such relief families may not be as able or willing to continue providing care for their aged relative.

5. To Serve as Bridges Between Institutional and Community-Based Care Systems. Case managers have the potential to serve as bridges between institutional and community-based care. If case managers are allowed to follow their clients through transitions—even as they enter and exit hospitals and nursing homes—they can assist hospital and nursing home discharge planners in facilitating patients' returns home. A case manager can discuss the available community care options with a client and his or her caregivers, and can help to develop and strengthen the client's informal support system until the client can readjust to living in the community.

Goals That Are Primarily System Oriented

1. To Facilitate the Development of a Broader Array of Noninstitutional Services. Care planning can be seen as a resource allocation activity. Case managers make important decisions about how much service clients will receive and from which providers. These care planning choices can close service gaps, facilitate the development of new services, and uncover costly duplications.

Awareness of local resources makes the case manager an authority on service gaps and overlap that exists in a community. Case managers may also affect the long-term care delivery system through program development and by fostering collaboration among providers. As opportunities arise to educate government officials, provider agencies, and funding agencies, case managers can testify expertly on the kinds of services that are needed at the community level.

2. To Promote Quality and Efficiency in the Delivery of Long-Term Care Services. In the same way that case managers have the capacity to facilitate the development of a broader array of noninstitutional services, they are in a unique position to affect the quality and efficiency of those services in the local delivery system. By working with providers and monitoring services that clients receive, case managers are able to evaluate the quality of providers' care. In the care planning process, case managers can also offer incentives to providers by directing the flow of referrals, thereby promoting both quality and efficiency.

3. To Enhance the Coordination of Long-Term Care Service Delivery. Case management is designed to enhance coordinated service delivery. For clients who are receiving several services, the case manager can be the central figure responsible for coordinating services and communicating with each client's multiple providers. Case managers strive to reduce service duplication that can occur when multiple providers each prepare separate care plans for the same client.

4. To Target Individuals Most at Risk of Nursing Home Placement in Order to Prevent Inappropriate Institutionalization. Case management has been proposed as a mechanism that can, in combination with community-based long-term care services, prevent inappropriate or premature institutionalization. In screening applicants, programs identify those clients who are "frail" and at risk of nursing home placement. In general, this so-called targeting is accomplished either by diverting individuals about to enter nursing homes to community-based services (preadmission screening) or by assessing individuals residing in the community for risk of institutionalization (nursing home certification) and arranging services where needed.

Accurate targeting can effect cost containment. It has been argued that long-term care costs can be reduced by targeting services to people at home who would have entered nursing homes if in-home care was not available.

5. To Contain Costs by Controlling Client Access to Services, Especially High-Cost Services. A case management agency's ability to contain costs depends not only on its success in targeting clients who are actually at risk of institutionalization, but also on developing lower cost community-based service packages and on paying for those services. Each function of case management supports the goal of assuring that services are appropriately utilized based on assessed need. Case managers serve as the initial screen for access to services. As they develop care plans, monitor, and reassess clients, they can provide needed services within fiscal constraints. Coale (1983) explained the dynamics of this system: "The conscious interplay between the subjective input from the case manager's contact with individual clients and the objectivity compelled by stressing cost effectiveness is the best way to provide compassionate service efficiently and at a reasonable cost" (p. 2).

In the absence of clear public policy directions for long-term care services, case management has been used as the primary means of achieving both client and system goals. But even though case management has enjoyed widespread acceptance, these goals are often contradictory. On the system side, case management can be inserted into ongoing delivery systems, and, depending on the kinds and amount of authority vested in the role, can be operational with minimal disruption of the existing delivery system. On the side of the client, however, case managers increasingly become change agents in their local delivery systems, as they gain more "gatekeeping" authority. They supply both the sanctions and incentives that shape provider behavior. Although case managers may have increased gatekeeping authority, they also continue to have responsibility for individual clients, including advocacy and counseling. While it may, in fact, be possible to be simultaneously the agent of the client and the agent of the system, case managers who try to accomplish both may experience considerable tension and stress. To handle that stress, they address multiple and conflicting goals on a daily basis by meeting one at a time, trying to resolve system and client conflicts simultaneously. Unless it is possible to argue that client and system goals are the same most of the time, case managers will continue to have difficulty successfully meeting all of the goals discussed above.

MODELS OF CASE MANAGEMENT

Case management models are distinguished primarily by the way they implement the plan of care (See Figure 1-1). Care planning is a resource allocation process. The care plan represents a prescription

Figure 1.1 Case Management Models.

CORE COMPONENTS		*MODELS*
• SCREENING		
• ASSESSMENT		
	⎧ • *resource allocation*	• *broker*
• *CARE PLANNING*	⎨ • *financing*	• *service management*
	⎩ • *authority*	• *managed care*
• PLAN IMPLEMENTATION		
• MONITORING		
• REASSESSMENT		

and a specification of services to be used by the client. The underlying structure of a program's financing has a fundamental impact on the kind of care planning provided. We have identified three major models of case management: broker, service management, and managed care.

The first case management model is called the *broker model*. Case managers who function as brokers do not have service dollars to spend on behalf of their clients. They develop care plans and they make referrals using services funded within the existing service delivery system. There is no guarantee that referrals made by case managers who operate as brokers will in fact be delivered.

The *service management* model of case management is based upon care planning that operates within specified fiscal limits. The funding source is the basis for a case manager's power to authorize services and her or his designation as the fiscally accountable person. In the service management model, case managers develop care plans within predetermined cost caps, usually a specified percentage of the cost of nursing home care. The service management model is found in the Home and Community-Based Waiver (2176) programs funded through Medicaid in 41 states.

The *managed care* model is the newest approach and is based on prospective financing. Prospective financing creates "provider risk" where financial responsibility and liability for expenditures are shifted to provider agencies. Providers are at risk for expenditures that exceed the prepaid amount and can create a surplus if costs are kept below capitated payments the agency receives. This puts additional pressure on the care planning process, creating incentives for the provider to control total costs, to provide and promote prevention oriented services, and to substitute lower cost services wherever possible without sacrificing quality or underserving clients.

The prevailing direction in the development of contemporary case management programs is toward more service management and managed care. As funding sources are structured to promote cost containment through prospective payment and target budgets, case managers will become more and more involved in accountability for fiscal decisions made during care planning and for aggregate costs in their programs and agencies. This is not to suggest that client advocacy will be overlooked, but that the case management job is becoming more complex, involving not only advocacy and service coordination, but also financial responsibility and gatekeeping functions.

BASIC PROGRAM COMPONENTS

There is no single definitive model of case management that can be incorporated into every delivery system. Beatrice (1981) has written:

> Case management is therefore neither inherently nor definitively defined. It derives its definition in large part from the nature and needs of a system whose component parts it will be coordinating and integrating. . .it must be a creature of its environment, tuned to the specific characteristics and needs of its host system, if it is to be effective (p. 124).

The program within which case management is embedded is ultimately more important for understanding how to structure the case management role than an analysis of case management variations in a vacuum. Variations in the way case management is implemented have their roots in four basic programmatic features: funding/reimbursement, targeting, gatekeeping, and organizational auspices (Austin, et al., 1985). These four dimensions describe the *programmatic goals and context* that define the case management function. Each of these dimensions is briefly introduced below, and discussed extensively in Chapter 3.

The foundation of long-term care service delivery is the underlying structure of its *funding/reimbursement*. As concern over long-term care costs mounts, various innovative financial approaches have been advanced, many of which represent alternatives to fee-for-service reimbursement. These include: caps on budgets (agency and client care plans), client cost sharing (copayments and deductibles), pooled funding (a feature of Social/HMO financing), case mix reimbursement formula, prepaid and capitated funding (tied to diagnosis as DRGs or to each enrollee as in Social/HMO), long-term care insurance, and continuing care retirement communities. Financing clearly affects the structure and function of case management.

Targeting involves the specification of subgroups within a population whose members are seen as the most appropriate recipients of services. For example, some community-based long-term care programs have targeted services to vulnerable, frail individuals, i.e. those persons "at risk" of nursing home placement. Outreach, screening, and assessment are central activities in the implementation of targeting, which is seen as a key element in controlling costs and possibly achieving savings.

Gatekeeping mechanisms are designed to control the number and types of clients or patients who have access to services, especially high-cost services such as institutional care. For example, nursing home preadmission screening efforts are designed to limit access to nursing home beds to frail individuals with multiple problems and functional deficits (i.e., elders who lack social supports, and who may reside in inappropriate housing). Gatekeeping also entails the implementation of specific budgetary limitations on the costs of service provision.

The fourth dimension of variation in case management is *organizational auspices*. What kinds of delivery systems should provide case management services? The choices here are expanding. Traditionally, case management has been provided by social service agencies; however, hospitals have recently started to provide the service. Other providers involved in case management include nursing homes, housing agencies, home health agencies, HMOs, and continuing care retirement communities. In some instances, independent agencies are created whose sole responsibility is providing case management services.

The preceding four dimensions must be clearly specified prior to undertaking the development of a case management service. This programmatic analysis will identify the parameters within which case managers will operate in a given program. The extent to which case managers have fiscal authority and are accountable for the care plans they design and implement represents the key defining characteristic of any case management model.

THE LARGER POLICY CONTEXT

The case management role represents only one component of the current structure of long-term care service delivery today (Kane & Kane, 1987). Case management, as a service, is constrained by fiscal, structural, environmental, and political realities and in itself represents one of several long-term care public policy initiatives. In order to be thoroughly understood, case management must be put into a larger public policy context. At the state level, this context encompasses states' Certificate of Need Programs, the supply of nursing home beds (ratio and absolute numbers), the rate of growth of the nursing home bed supply, and the nature of any preadmission screening program that is operational. This kind of comparative analysis provides a broader perspective on case management in community-based long-term care programs (Applebaum, Austin, & Atchley, 1987).

Certificate of Need—Certificate of Need (CON) programs are state regulatory mechanisms exercised by health planning agencies to review and approve capital expenditures and service capacity expansions by hospitals, nursing homes, and other health care facilities. In a state with CON, a health care facility may not undertake a reviewable project unless it obtains planning agency approval based on a finding of community need. States adopted CON to achieve various policy goals, foremost among which was controlling health care costs by restricting the growth of institutional health services. CON programs were intended to substitute regulatory controls for weak market restraints on expansion and new technology introduction in the health care sector. Cost containment is not, however, the only goal of CON state regulation. States have also pursued goals associated with quality of care, geographic distribution of facilities, and subsidizing indigent care. "The great majority of states seem to have originally established CON programs to balance multiple, and sometimes competing goals relating to cost, quality and accessibility of health services" (Simpson, 1985, p. 1).

Nursing Home Bed Supply—The availability of nursing home beds represents an important component in the provision of long-term care services in any state. States have varied widely in terms of how much they have invested in institutional long-term care services. A review of the ratio of nursing home beds to population over age 65 and the actual number of beds in 1978 and 1983 across states shows that 29 states experienced a decrease in the ratio of beds to population during this interval, while only four experienced a decrease in actual beds, reflecting the growth of the population over age 65. On average, during this period, the ratio decreased by 2.8%; however, the actual number of beds increased by 10.2%.

Preadmission Screening—An increasing number of states have developed preadmission screening (PAS) programs to evaluate nursing home applicants prior to admission. The purpose of these programs is to assure that nursing home placement is needed and appropriate. Both the number and scope of these programs have grown considerably in the last decade as states attempt to reduce inappropriate placements and control nursing home costs and utilization.

A recent national survey by Interstudy located 31 PAS programs operating in 29 states and the District of Columbia. Over two-thirds of these programs operate on a statewide basis. In 90% of states with screening, PAS is required before Medicaid will reimburse nursing home or community-based services. Fifteen programs reported that they coordinate, provide, or fund community-based services in conjunction with PAS. Programs are operated through a wide variety of state aging and Medicaid agencies. At the local level, there is also considerable variation. Public agencies represent the bulk of organizations administering the program, although 19% of the states reported the use of contracting to private agencies for a portion of the process. Interstudy researchers found that "within each state, there seem to be at least some territorial conflict between components of the long-term care system concerning what organization should be responsible for conducting PAS. In some cases, states appear to believe strongly that PAS should be conducted by a disinterested public or private health/human service agency. This sort of screening is perceived to be objective and therefore in the best interest of the client" (Interstudy, 1986, p. 67).

The target population to be screened shows some variation across the country. Ten programs reported screening only Medicaid eligible persons (in eight of these 10 states this was mandated by state law). Six states require screening of both the Medicaid and spend down populations. Fifteen programs state that all nursing home applications may or must be screened, with screening mandatory for those eligible for Medicaid. Three of these 15 states (Indiana, Minnesota, and New Jersey) require screening for both Medicaid and private pay nursing home applicants.

Choices made regarding the nature of the Section 2176 Medicaid waiver program, CON efforts, nursing home bed supply, PAS program, and reimbursement issues (not discussed here) represent the components of state-level public policy for long-term care service delivery. A thorough analysis of public policy for long-term care in any state must start with a comprehensive view of the pieces that make up this complex set of relationships. Among them are the supply of both institutional and community-based services, public demand for and expectations regarding care, gatekeeping mechanisms to control access to costly services, incentives built into the reimbursement system that may favor the development of one part of the delivery system over others, and creative utilization of multiple funding streams and the interrelationships among these.

WHY DOES EVERYONE WANT TO DO CASE MANAGEMENT?

Growth in the availability of case management services has been accompanied by considerable controversy over the most appropriate organizational location, professional group, and/or programmatic affiliation for the service. Discussions have focused on the appropriateness of providing case management from a free standing case management/planning organization or through a provider agency; by nurses or social workers; in health or social service agencies, and so forth. Since the core case management tasks represent, in the most generalizable and abstract case, good professional practice with attention to comprehensive assessment, continuity of care, monitoring, and reassessment, it would be difficult to find a human service professional group that did not claim to perform case management tasks. From this point of view, physicians have also claimed to be case managers.

Beyond the foundation of case management in professional practice, there is another factor motivating the widespread interest in case management. Providers understand that case management will be provided in those locations that are designated as delivery system entry points. Identifying and screening potential clients is the first step in a sequence of case management activities that includes care planning and plan implementation. These tasks are resource allocation and distribution activities. Indirectly through referral or directly through purchase of service, case managers function as resource allocators and distributors in their local delivery systems. As such, case managers potentially function with considerable power and authority. It is not hard to understand why providers and professional groups claim to be case managers and vie for the resource designation. As case management moves out of the broker category and into the service management and managed care categories, we can anticipate even greater competition for the case management function.

Chapter 2

Components of Case Management

Despite the different models and approaches to implementing managed care, case management has a common set of core components that include: 1) outreach, 2) screening or intake and eligibility determination, 3) formalized assessment, 4) care planning, 5) service arrangement, 6) ongoing monitoring and follow-up, and 7) formalized reassessment. In the description that follows, these basic components of the case management process will be defined and the rationale for their development examined. To help provide an overview of the core case management components we will draw upon the experiences of 16 long-term care demonstration projects. These projects, implemented between 1973 and 1985, were designed to test the use of case management in conjunction with an expanded array of community based services. These studies (See Table 2–1) provide a wealth of information about the provision of case management, although the studies were not generally designed to test different approaches to case management.

OUTREACH/IDENTIFYING THE TARGET POPULATION

Outreach activities include efforts to publicize the services offered by an agency and to identify persons likely to qualify for and need case management. "Casefinding" and "locating the target population" are other terms for outreach. Older persons experiencing high levels of

TABLE 2–1 Demonstration Strategies: Long-Term Care Projects

I. Develop, coordinate, and upgrade long-term care delivery system	
Worcester Home Care	1973–1975
Wisconsin CCO	1973–1979
Triage I & II	1974–1979
Alternative Health Services—Georgia	1976–1981
Washington Community-Based Care	1976–1978
California MSSP	1980–1984
Florida Pentastar	1980–1982
New York City Home Care	1980–1983
New York's Nursing Home Without Walls	1980–Present
Financial Control Channeling	1982–1985
Project Open	1980–1983
San Diego Long-Term Care	1981–1984
II. Control client access to and utilization of institutional services	
ACCESS I & II	1975–Present
Texas ICF II	1980–1985
South Carolina LTCP	1980–1984
III. Consolidate long-term care service delivery into a single agency	
A. On Lok (final phase) and Expansion Sites	9/71–Present
B. S/HMO	1985–Present

disability may have the most difficulty gaining access to services. As a result, outreach efforts help to locate these persons and connect them with appropriate services. Outreach mechanisms can include: being listed with an information and referral agency; making agreements with provider agencies to make referrals to the case management agency; public information campaigns; and being part of a nursing home preadmission screening process. Outreach activities reflect the targeting requirement of the case management program and thus represent the first step toward reaching the program's target population.

SCREENING

Screening is a preliminary assessment of clients' circumstances and resources that is done to determine presumptive eligibility and appropriateness for a case management program. In many programs, screening criteria are used to target those clients at risk of institutionalization. For example, in the National Long-Term Care Channeling Demonstration, the largest of the demonstration projects implemented in 10 states, functional disability, cognitive or behavioral problems affecting functioning, unmet needs for care, and the existence of a fragile informal support system were the criteria used to identify applicants likely to need nursing home care (Applebaum, 1988). These criteria were applied to determine whether the clients' needs and circumstances matched the target population definition of the program. As such, the screening function is a key step in targeting services to the appropriate population.

A standard instrument that is considerably shorter than a comprehensive assessment is generally used to screen potential applicants. The screening process is designed so that only those clients whose needs and circumstances appear to meet the program's eligibility criteria receive the more lengthy and costly comprehensive assessment. This can be accomplished through a variety of techniques including written referrals, telephone reviews, or in-person screenings. Use of the telephone seems to be a common mode in many programs and demonstrations as it is more friendly than written referrals, but less costly than in-person screens. The National Channeling Demonstration was typical in its approach, administering a standardized instrument over the telephone. The Channeling sites completed each screen in 15 or 20 minutes, on average, generally using paraprofessional staff. This was consistent with the experience of other demonstrations. In the 13 long-term care demonstration projects reviewed in a study by the Berkeley Planning Associates (BPA) (Haskins et al., 1985), the screening step was viewed as the least professionalized of the case management functions, and was typically performed by clerical staff or persons with diverse undergraduate training.

COMPREHENSIVE ASSESSMENT

Comprehensive assessment is "a method of collecting in-depth information about a person's social situation and physical, mental and psychological functioning which allows identification of the person's problems and care needs in the major functional areas" (Schneider & Weiss, p. 12 1982; Burack-Weiss, 1988). As such, it functions as both a targeting mechanism and as a first step in the service allocation process. The areas commonly evaluated in the comprehensive assessment include: physical health; mental functioning (both cognitive and affective); ability to perform activities of daily living; social supports; physical environment of the home; and financial resources. Because frail elderly have multiple health problems, functional disabilities, and social losses, many experts believe that a comprehensive multidimensional assessment is required for effective care planning and service arrangement.

Comprehensive assessments are generally performed for every client who is screened into the program. The assessment interview is conducted in person, usually in the client's home. Family members are typically interviewed as well to assess the client's informal support system and the family's ability and desire to provide care to the client.

Standard instruments are most often used in the assessment process. For example, the Sickness Impact Profile (SIP) and the Older Americans Resource Survey (OARS) instrument are multidimensional assessment tools designed to measure capacity in all functional areas. Some programs have designed their own instruments and/or have combined other less comprehensive standardized tools that focus on specific domains of assessment (e.g., the Mental Status Questionnaire [MSQ] to measure cognitive functioning; the Beck Depression Index to measure affective functioning; and the Katz ADL and Lawton & Brody IADL to measure ability to perform the activities and instrumental activities of daily living) into a multidimensional instrument. Table 2–2 outlines the types of assessment instruments used by 16 long-term care projects.

TABLE 2–2 Assessment Instruments Used in Long-Term Care Projects*

Project	Instruments
1. Wisconsin CCO	OARS Areas of Care Evaluation Instrument Quality of Life Instrument Grauer Scale
2. Triage, Connecticut	ADL IADL MSQ "Triage Quality of Life Index" "Triage Assessment & Reassessment Form"
3. AHS—Georgia	"Client Assessment Interview" developed by AHS
4. Washington Community-Based Care	OARS
5. ACCESS (Monroe County Long-Term Care Program)	"Patient Assessment Form" developed by ACCESS

TABLE 2–2 Assessment Instruments Used in Long-Term Care Projects*

Project	Instruments
6. On Lok, San Francisco	Interdisciplinary team assessment
7. FIG/Waiver, Oregon	"Patient Information Base" (PIB) (a functional assessment tool developed by the state)
8. New York's Nursing Home Without Walls	New York State's DMS-1 assessment form
9. Texas ICF—II	Comprehensive assessment instrument developed by the state
10. Project OPEN, Mt. Zion Hospital, San Francisco	"Functional Status Instrument" included: ADL IADL MSQ
11. South Carolina Long-Term Care Project	Comprehensive assessment instrument developed by state
12. Home Care Project, New York City	New York State's DMS-1 assessment form "Physician Summary" (completed by client's physician)
13. Pentastar Project, Florida	Client Assessment Form 3003 (used throughout Florida for Aging & Adult Services clients) "Comprehensive Medical Assessment" developed for Pentastar Short Portable MSQ
14. Allied Home Health Services, North San Diego County	Philadelphia Geriatric Morale Scale ADL MSQ other client assessment instruments developed by the project
15. M.S.S.P., California	ADL IADL MSQ
16. National Long-Term Care Channeling Demonstration	"Hybrid" clinical-research baseline assessment instrument (developed for the project; built on several existing functional assessment instruments)

The use of standardized multidimensional assessment instruments is the state-of-the-art in long-term care assessment. Considerable attention has been paid to developing instruments that accurately assess the major functional areas of an older person's well-being. Standardization has enabled researchers to compare and analyze data gathered from large numbers of clients across programs and projects. In this chapter, we will not discuss the various issues raised relating to the selection of appropriate assessment instruments. Several major works (Kane & Kane, 1981; George & Landerman, 1982; Phillips, 1981) have provided a comprehensive discussion of assessment instruments, procedures, and their specific applications.

Trained professionals either individually or as part of a team typically conducted the comprehensive assessments. Assessment teams, composed of a registered nurse and a social worker, were the most common configuration. Individual professionals, generally a nurse or social worker with cross-discipline review, is the next most common approach. Select projects (The ACCESS project in New York, and the Florida Pentastar program) contracted out for part or all of the assessment for select clients.

CARE PLANNING

Care planning is the process by which information gathered during assessment is translated into a package of services (Schneider, 1988). It is a resource allocation process where a service prescription is written for a client. Care planning can be performed by a single case manager or in team care planning conferences. Care planning functions in the majority of long-term care demonstrations were completed by interdisciplinary team members who typically possessed either professional or advanced professional degrees. Four projects—Georgia AHS, MSSP, Triage, and Wisconsin CCO—involved nonprofessional staff in the care planning team. Subsequently, these staff had responsibility for arranging services and/or monitoring following care planning. In the Channeling demonstration, care plans were prepared by the case manager, but were subject to supervisory and/or peer review.

The *Channeling Case Management Manual* notes that "care planning is that portion of the case management process which calls for the greatest amount of clinical judgment, creativity and sensitivity" (Schneider & Weiss, p. 27 1982). Through care planning, the case manager also performs an important resource allocation function. A service prescription is written. The care plan identifies services that are going to be used by a client and will no longer be available in the community delivery system if, in fact, they are used by that client.

Financing that underlies the program in which a case manager works fundamentally shapes the nature of the care planning process. A case manager who is working in a 2176 Waiver program (Home- and Community-Based Medicaid Waivers), functions very differently than a case manager who writes care plans in a program financed exclusively by Title III of the Older Americans Act. The primary difference is that in the waiver program case managers have purchase power in the form of service dollars to spend on behalf of the client, while in the Title III program case managers primarily make referrals. They have direct access only to providers under contract with the Older Americans Act funds. Case managers who function as brokers write care plans and make referrals. There is no guarantee, however, that those referrals will result in service delivery. The broker case manager has no clout and no leverage with providers. The broker acts as an advocate on behalf of the client, attempting to increase providers' responsiveness to his or her clients' needs, but there is no way the broker can guarantee service provision.

A key issue is whether the care plans are systematically costed out. Do case managers know what they are spending? What is the breadth of services case managers can buy and how broad is their involvement in the delivery system? For case managers in service management or managed care models, the selection of an array of services for his or her clients, as outlined in the care plan, has significant cost implications. Case managers operating within specific budgetary limits must be able to judge when a client's community or in-home care plan will exceed the cost of providing a comparable level of care in a nursing home. Case managers' skill in making these choices and estimates is an important factor in controlling long-term care costs (Rickards, 1983).

Involvement of clients' informal caregivers is also an essential part of the care planning process. The goal is to negotiate feasible informal support in combination with formally provided services. The case manager can assist in stimulating and enhancing clients' independent functioning and supporting clients' caregivers. Caregiver support services may become a significant component of the care plan. The case manager may be able to identify new sources of informal support, and strengthen existing sources by expanding the support network. Case managers often find that clients are referred when their caregivers have reached the point of "burnout." In these cases, the case manager's client is both the older person and her or his primary caregiver.

SERVICE ARRANGEMENT

The service arrangement function of case management is a process of contacting both formal and informal providers to arrange for services outlined in the care plan. Service arrangement and plan implementation involve negotiating with providers for services that both meet clients' needs and are cost effective. Service arrangement also distributes resources to providers in the local delivery system. The service arrangement process is simplified when agreements have previously been established between the case management agency and providers, either informally or through formal written agreements such as a memorandum of understanding (Johnson & Sterthous, 1982).

A key aspect of service arrangement involves sharing client assessment and care plan information with all relevant informal and formal providers. Gottesman, Ishizaki, & MacBride (1979) noted the value of this activity while implementing a case management program in Pennsylvania Area Agencies on Aging. Although families provided 80% of all service the clients received, family members were not informed about what formal services would be provided to their parent or what they were expected to do as part of the care plan. In addition, physicians were seldom informed regarding how the services they had ordered would be provided. As a result, persons involved in care plan decisionmaking were not adequately informed.

MONITORING

Monitoring is "the continuing contact the case manager has with providers and clients to ensure that services are provided in accordance with the care plan and to ascertain whether these services continue to meet the client's needs" (Schneider & Weiss, p. 36 1982). Monitoring is a critical case management task that enables the case manager to respond quickly to changes in the client's status and increase, decrease, terminate, or maintain services as indicated. Responsiveness to changes in clients' needs can have a dramatic impact on service costs. The frequency of monitoring varies depending on the intensity of client needs and the type of services being delivered. For example, a client who has just been discharged from the hospital after an acute illness and is temporarily receiving home health care from two shifts of in-home workers may need substantial monitoring. Occasional monitoring may be all that is required by a client who is stable and receiving meals and weekly personal care.

The level of staff professionalization in monitoring was similar to the staffing requirements of service arrangement in the demonstration projects. In projects where paraprofessional staff generally performed the monitoring function, clients who were in crisis situations or whose circumstances were more complex were referred to the more highly professionalized staff. BPA researchers concluded that it was unclear whether monitoring could be managed entirely by paraprofessional staff without access to professional staff for consultation and assistance. Channeling researchers, however, reported that monitoring was more time-consuming and challenging for project staff than they had originally anticipated (Carcagno, Applebaum, Christianson, Phillips, Thornton et al., 1986).

REASSESSMENT

Reassessment is the "scheduled or event-precipitated examination of the client's situation and functioning to identify changes which occurred since the initial or most recent assessment and to measure progress toward the desired outcomes outlined in the care plan" (Schneider & Weiss, 1982). Reassessment in research and demonstration projects included regularly scheduled readministering of all or part of the original assessment instrument. In research projects, this was done for data collection purposes as dictated by the research design. In nonresearch programs, reassessment tended to be a partial reevaluation of the most significant client problems. Often, reassessment dates are written into the care plan based upon the case manager's judgment of an appropriate time frame.

Timing of reassessment in research projects varied. In the National Long-Term Care Channeling Demonstration, the first reassessment occurred after three months, then every six months thereafter. Of the long-term care demonstration projects reviewed by BPA, eight administered reassessments every six months (Triage, Georgia AHS, Wisconsin CCO, On Lok, Washington Community-Based Care, San Diego, New York City Home Care Project, Project OPEN). Three projects performed reassessments every three months (North San Diego County Community Long-Term Care Project, Wisconsin CCO-Milwaukee, South Carolina Community Long-Term Care Project). Finally, one project, ACCESS, reassessed clients every four months.

Reassessments were also performed in the Channeling project when a major event in a client's life triggered a full reassessment. The events that triggered reassessment included loss of a major caretaker through death or relocation; death of a client's spouse or member of the household; acute medical crisis; major deterioration in physical or mental status; placement in a hospital or nursing home; and forced relocation of the client. If the relocation substantially changed the care plan by moving the client away from neighbors who formerly provided informal support, a reassessment was indicated. Reassessment can be triggered by other events as well; such as when the initial problem had been resolved, alleviated, or redefined; when planned service was discontinued by the service provider or the client; or when there was a planned withdrawal of a service and a need to help the client see this change positively. In other cases, reassessment may result in termination. The agency may want to terminate services to clients who have improved or stabilized in order to make way for new, waiting clients. Finally, reassessment may be conducted when a new worker is assigned to the case (Steinberg & Carter, 1983).

Whether performed at regularly scheduled intervals or on an as-needed basis, reassessments often result in changes in care plans. This final step creates a feedback loop that makes case management an ongoing process. Altered care plans require implementation and monitoring just as initial care plans did. Changes in a care plan can be significant, reflecting major disrupting events in clients' lives, or care plan changes may be minor, resulting in modifications of the types and intensity of services delivered. From a programmatic perspective, reassessment can significantly alter program costs. It is a major gatekeeping function.

Staffing of reassessment mirrors staffing patterns for the initial assessment process. In all 13 projects reviewed by BPA, reassessments were performed by the same staff who conducted the initial assessment. If these individuals were not available, the reassessment was conducted by staff with a similar level of professionalization.

This review demonstrates the extent to which the implementation of case management varied across demonstration projects. No one approach to case management service delivery has been demonstrated to be superior to the others; however, consensus does exist regarding the core case management components.

Chapter 3

How Program Variables Affect Case Management Service Delivery

In order to thoroughly comprehend how a program influences the limits within which case managers perform, it is useful to analyze the programmatic context within which case management services are provided. The four major variables that affect the programmatic context are: financing/reimbursement, mechanisms, targeting criteria, gatekeeping, and organizational auspices (see Table 3–1). Each of these components is examined in the pages that follow.

FINANCING/REIMBURSEMENT MECHANISMS

The present funding system is fragmented. It is a fee-for-service system that allows providers to charge the service costs directly to the various programs for which the client is eligible. Fragmentation makes it difficult to control costs and hold any single provider accountable for the total costs associated with the care plan. Case managers are likely to control only a portion of the resources for any given client. The following financing strategies attempt to reduce these and other problems.

TABLE 3–1 Program Context Variables

Financing Reimbursement

—the financial basis of the program. Source, form, and amount of funding.
  Examples: pooled funding
              client cost sharing
              capitated/prospective funding
              waivers
              fee for service

Targeting Criteria

—the definition of the target population. Through targeting criteria, programs specify the type of client to be served and those who will not be served.
  Examples: "at risk of nursing home placement"
              ICF/SNF certified
              functionally impaired
              impaired cognitive functioning
              major loss or crisis
              unmet needs
              fragile informal support system

Gatekeeping

—gatekeeping mechanisms designed to control the number and types of services that clients have access to, particularly high cost services like institutional care. Closely related to targeting.
  Examples: authorization power
              cap on average expenditures
              cap on individual expenditures
              provider risk
              centralized authorization

Organizational Auspices

—the organizational location for case management activities.
  Examples: provider agency
              freestanding case management agency
              hospital
              adult day care center
              state/local agency
              private insurance company
              Health Maintenance Organization
              fee for service program/practitioner

Pooled and Prospective Funding

One mechanism used to reduce the fragmentation between funding sources involves the establishment of a funding pool. This pooled funding idea is designed to control costs, by supporting interagency coordination and helping case managers make better matches between clients' needs and services, thus reducing fragmentation among programs.

Pooled funding is designed to facilitate cost control by fixing in advance the maximum amount of long-term care funds that will be available for the caseload. In the National Channeling Demonstration, pooled funds were provided in the amount of 60 percent of the average local Medicaid rates for SNF and ICF care for the aggregate caseload. Medicare paid 60 percent of that amount, and Medicaid, state, and local funds contributed the remaining 40 percent. Such an approach has been used in several of the long-term care demonstrations.

The Social/HMO also incorporates a funds pool including revenue from Medicare, Medicaid, private premiums, and client cost sharing. Medicare and Medicaid rates involve adjustments for case mix. "Each site repeatedly reviewed revenue and cost assumptions and reconsidered its decisions on such issues as premium levels, long-term care benefit structure, utilizations assumptions, eligibility criteria and related case mix assumptions" (Leutz, Greenberg, Abrahams, Pruttas, Diamond, & Gruenberg, 1985, p. 215). However, the Social/HMO tests a new concept, a prospective and capitated payment system. This reimbursement system represents a major departure from the fee-for-service funding approach. Providers prospectively receive a fixed amount per client. Capitated funding for medical and long-term care services is also being tested in the On Lok program. Both are consolidated models of long-term care delivery systems incorporating acute, ambulatory, and long-term care services. The primary difference between the two demonstrations is their target populations. On Lok serves only a nursing home certifiable population, while Social/HMO enrollees are a representative population of elders (well, moderately impaired, and frail).

Results from On Lok are encouraging. Its success indicates that cost savings may have been achieved, at least partially, through the application of prepaid funding (Haskins, et al., 1985). Preliminary indications from the Social/HMO suggest that effective case management and targeting have kept costs within the limits imposed by the pooled/capitated approach. These projects represent promising financing and service delivery approaches that promote higher levels of integration through innovative funding, provider risk, and care provision strategies, although final research results are not yet available.

The use of pooled funding has received some attention at the national policy level. Some have recommended the creation of a new federal program that would combine the long-term care provision of Medicare, Medicaid, the Social Services Block Grant (Title XX), and Title III of the Older Americans Act (Callahan, 1981). Initially, this program would review state plans, but eventually it would also fund block grants. Other proposals, such as the bill proposed by the late Congressman Claude Pepper, advocate expanding Medicare so that it will provide community-based long-term care benefits.

Client Cost Sharing

In order to target public funds to clients with limited incomes, clients with higher incomes have been asked to share in the cost of their services. Client cost sharing was used in three long-term care projects: ACCESS, New York's Nursing Home Without Walls, and Channeling. In the financial control model of the Channeling Demonstration, clients whose incomes exceeded a protected amount (200 percent of the state's supplementary income eligibility level and a food stamp bonus) were required to contribute to partially cover the costs of their services. Clients were not asked to pay for services they would ordinarily receive at no cost, nor were they required to pay more than the cost of the services received.

Cost sharing, or co-insurance, is a key feature of the Social/HMO. Given the provider risk feature of this demonstration, client cost sharing plays a key part in managing revenue and allocation patterns. Leutz, et al. (1985) suggested that the range of mechanisms Social/HMO sites have adopted for structuring client co-insurance can be used to affect both demand for long-term care services and the distribution of chronic care benefits among project enrollees.

TARGETING CRITERIA

The specification of targeting criteria is a major component of any case management program. Although most demonstration projects attempted to target their scarce resources to frail individuals at risk of nursing home placement, the record indicates that their capacity to accurately target this group has been mixed. In most of the long-term care demonstrations, few clients in either the experimental or control groups actually entered nursing homes (Haskins, et al., 1984; Kemper, et al., 1987). The exception to this general trend was South Carolina's Community Long-Term Care Project, which required nursing home preadmission screening. Clients entering this program were both applying for and certified eligible for a nursing home level of care. This experience suggests that current long-term care assessment technology may not adequately capture the complex variables that predict likelihood of nursing home admission, although it can identify persons whose disabilities and living conditions indicate the need for a nursing home level of care (Capitman, Haskins, & DeGraaf, 1983). Another difficulty is that many extremely frail elders residing in the community may functionally resemble nursing home residents, but may not be actively seeking nursing home care (Weissert, 1985a). The accuracy of targeting directly affects program costs, especially if community-based services are viewed as substitutes for nursing home care.

Table 3–2 displays the targeting criteria used by 20 long-term care demonstration projects. Some criteria are objective, e.g., residence, age, and Medicare or Medicaid eligibility. Other criteria are verifiable, e.g., "ICF/SNF certified" or "about to be discharged from a hospital or nursing home." Some criteria, however, are more subjective and require professional judgment to interpret assessment data. For example, a case manager may have to determine the extent to which a client meets a given criteria such as "requires assistance with personal care," "frailty of the informal support system," or "is at risk of institutional placement." The more commonly used targeting criteria are discussed in the sections that follow.

Certification for Nursing Home Level of Care

The most restrictive targeting criteria are found in programs that define client eligibility in terms of being ICF/SNF (Intermediate or Skilled Care) certified or "certifiable." Five long-term care demonstrations utilized this eligibility criterion: South Carolina, ACCESS, Georgia's AHS, On Lok, and Nursing Home Without Walls (Kemper, et al., 1987). Targeting is also a central feature of the Medicaid (2176) Home and Community-Based Waiver Program. Under the waiver, states are to provide care to those who would otherwise be in nursing homes. The Social/HMO demonstration also uses nursing home certification to determine eligibility for chronic care services.

An increasing number of states have developed preadmission screening programs (PAS) to evaluate nursing home applicants prior to admission. Both the number and scope of these programs have grown considerably in the last decade as states attempt to reduce

TABLE 3–2 Targeting Criteria of Long-Term Care Projects

PROJECTS

Targeting Criteria	Wisconsin CCO	Triage	Triage II	Georgia AHS	WA-Community Based Care	ACCESS	On Lok	OR-FIG/Waiver	Texas ICF II	NY-Nursing Homes Without Walls	Project OPEN	South Carolina CLTCP	NY-Home Care Project	Florida-Pentastar	San Diego LTCP	MSSP	Channeling-Basic	Channeling-Financial	2176 Waiver	S/HMO (LTC Benefit)
Residence	X	X	X	X	X	X	X	X	X	X	X	X	X	X	X	X	X	X		
Age	18	65	65	50	18	18	55	65	18	any age	65	18	65	60	65	65	65	65	18+	65
Medicare eligible		X		X		X		X		X	X	X		X			X		X	
Medicaid eligible	X			X	X		10%		X	X		X		X		X			X	
ICF/SNF Certified				X	X	X	X		X	X		X							X	X
At risk of nursing home placement	X		X	X	X	X				X	X			X	X	X				
Functionally impaired/Needs ADL/IADL assist	X		X	X	X	X					X	X	X	X	X	X	X	X	X	X
Mental functioning problems						X							X	X			X	X		
Community-based care plan cost limit				X	X			X		X		X				X		X	X	X
Major loss or crisis											X					X	X	X		

32

Unmet needs/fragile informal support system											X	X	X			
Potential for/About to be discharged from nursing home	X	X	X	X	X					X			X			
About to be discharged from hospital	X		X	X	X					X			X	X	X	
Recently hospitalized							X		X	X			X			
At the risk of frequent hospital admissions	X					X			X	X			X			
Lack of community services	X								X							
Monitoring and education needed to maintain stable state	X	X							X							

33

inappropriate placements and control nursing home costs and utilization.

A recent national survey by Interstudy (1986) located 31 PAS programs operating in 29 states and the District of Columbia. Over two thirds of the programs operate on a statewide basis. In 90% of the preadmission programs, PAS is required before Medicaid will reimburse nursing home or community-based services. Fifteen programs reported that they coordinate, provide, or fund community-based services in conjunction with PAS. Programs are operated through a variety of public agencies (Aging and Medicaid) at state and local levels. The target population for screening varies across states as well. Ten states require screening for current Medicaid eligibles only. Another six states screen both current Medicaid clients as well as those who would spend down to Medicaid eligibility within a specified period. Fifteen state PAS programs screen all nursing home applicants, with optional screening for private paying clients but mandatory screening for Medicaid eligibles. Only three states (Indiana, Minnesota, and New Jersey) have instituted mandatory screening for *all* nursing home applicants (private pay, spend down, and Medicaid eligibles.)

At Risk of Nursing Home Placement

Some programs did not require formal certification of need for ICF/SNF level of care, but did target clients at risk of nursing home placement. Additional targeting criteria were often added to "at risk of nursing home placement." This included criteria such as "requires assistance with personal care," "at risk of frequent hospital admissions," "fragile informal support system." Assessing clients for risk of nursing home placement was usually based on a combination of formal assessment and professional judgment.

Considerable research has been conducted to identify factors that predict risk of institutionalization. In addition to functional disability, the following risk factors have been identified: older age (75); unmarried or widowed; being female; living in poverty; personal care dependency; living alone; mental disorientation; and having a high-risk medical problem such as cancer or digestive, blood, metabolic, genito-urinary, and circulatory disorders (Branch & Jette, 1982; Palmore, 1976; Weissert & Scanlon, 1983). By using these as operational targeting criteria, programs can theoretically identify persons who are the most likely to enter nursing homes.

The problem in identifying "high risk" individuals is essentially one of selecting assessment criteria that constitute "risk of nursing home placement." The eligibility criteria used in the Channeling Project (see Table 3–3) illustrate one approach to defining "risk of nursing home placement" in targeting criteria. Because previous long-term care demonstrations had reported difficulties identifying those clients at risk of nursing home placement, planners in the Channeling Dem-

TABLE 3–3 National Long-Term Care Channeling Demonstration Program Eligibility Criteria

	Explanation of criteria
Age	Must be 65 or over
Residence	Must reside within project catchment area; must be living in community or (if institutionalized) certified as likely to be discharged within three months.
Functional Disability	Must have two moderate impairments of functioning in activities of daily living (ADL), or three severe impairments of functioning in instrumental activities of daily living (IADL), or two severe IADL impairments and one severe ADL impairment.[a]
(Cognitive or Behavioral Problems Affecting Functioning)	(Cognitive or behavioral difficulties affecting individual ability to perform activities of daily living can count as one of the severe IADL impairments.)
Unmet Needs	Must need help with at least two categories of services affected by functional impairments for six months (meals, housework/shopping, medications, medical treatments at home, personal care).
(Fragile support)	(A fragile informal support system that may no longer be able to provide needed services can satisfy the unmet service needs criterion.)
Insurance Coverage	Must be Medicare Part A eligible (for the financial control model).

[a]The six ADL activities include bathing, dressing, toileting, transfer, continence, and eating. The seven IADL activities include housekeeping, shopping, meal preparation, taking medicine, travel, using the telephone, and managing finances. For the purpose of the IADL criterion, the first two and the last three IADLs were aggregated into two combined categories. Thus, there are four possible IADL areas in which applicants can qualify, plus the cognitive/behavioral impairment category which counts as one IADL item.

Source: From Baxter, R.J., Applebaum, R., Callahan Jr., J.J., Christianson, J.B., Day, S.L.: *The Planning and Implementation of Channeling: Early Experiences of the National Long Term Care Demonstration* (Princeton, NJ: Mathematica Policy Research), April 15, 1983, p. 114.

onstration spent considerable effort developing entry criteria. However, results from the Channeling study indicate that while the project succeeded in serving an extremely frail group of clients, a relatively small percentage (about 15% after 12 months) actually entered nursing homes (Kemper, et al., 1986).

Functionally Impaired/Needs Assistance with Activities of Daily Living and Instrumental Activities of Daily Living

Functional disability was a basic eligibility requirement for many case management demonstration projects, although the specific language used to define "functionally disabled" differed across programs.

Functional impairment criteria were operationalized by measuring need for assistance with both activities of daily living (ADLs) and instrumental activities of daily living (IADLs). For example, one criterion used by the San Diego Long-Term Care Demonstration project asked, "Is the client unable to maintain self at home without assistance in the activities of daily living?" In Project OPEN, one criterion used was "judged by interviewer to have difficulty with independent living."

Mental Functioning

Impairments in cognitive capacity may also affect client ADL and IADL functioning. Three long-term care demonstration projects (MSSP, New York City's Home Care Project, and Channeling) included mental impairment among their targeting criteria. Project OPEN required that clients' cognitive functioning be adequate to answer the questions on the assessment instrument.

An interesting problem in assessing mental impairment using ADL and IADL scales arose in the Channeling project. Channeling screening staff and referral sources reported that some individuals were inappropriately excluded from the project because mental functioning was not given enough importance as an entry criteria. Staff members expressed concern that behaviors associated with mental disorders, such as wandering, forgetfulness, and emotional conflicts, were not adequately weighted in the targeting criteria. Staff members found that "because individuals with mental disorders could in many cases perform physical activities of daily living independently, it was difficult for these applicants to meet program eligibility guidelines" (Baxter, Applebaum, Callahan, Christianson, & Day, 1983). The point here is that physical capacity to carry out activities of daily living can mask other functional deficits.

Community-Based Care Plan Cost Limitations

Nine projects (Georgia's AHS; ACCESS; South Carolina; Oregon's FIG/Waiver; MSSP; Channeling Financial Control Model; and New York's Nursing Home Without Walls, S/HMO, and 2176 Waiver projects) required that the cost of caring for clients in the community must be less than a designated percentage of the cost of nursing home care. Table 3–4 displays information on individual client cost

TABLE 3–4 Project Financial Caps

Project	Monthly cap (percent)	Monthly maximum with approval (percent)	Length of time exceeded before approval needed (months)	Approval authority
Access	75	110	not specified	Monroe Co. Dept. of Social Serv.
S. Carolina CLTC	75	200	not specified	Project Director
Oregon FIG/Waiver	75	not specified	3	Oregon Adult Family Service
AHS-Georgia	85 (80 serv. units/mo)	100 serv. units/mo	9	AHS Proj. Director
MSSP	70	105	1	Site Case Mgmt. Supervisor State Prog. Administrator
New York Nursing Home Without Walls	75	cannot exceed		
Channeling-Financial Control Model	85/client 60/entire proj. caseload	not specified	not specified	State approval
2176	varies by state	varies by state	varies by state	varies by state
S/HMO	$6250–12,000 max. annual benefit varies by state	same as cap	not specified	C.M. Supervisor

limitations for each project. Kemper, et al. (1987) reported that cost caps ranged from 60 to 85 percent of nursing home costs. Case managers could, however, fund some care plans that exceeded the cost limitation if it was anticipated that care plan costs would decrease over time. The S/HMO demonstration and the 2176 Home and Community-Based Waiver program also included a cost control component.

Developing care plans within specific budgetary limits serves several purposes. First, the process helps to identify persons whose care at home is too costly and who might more appropriately be admitted to nursing homes. Second, care plan cost parameters require case managers to develop plans very carefully. As a result, over time, case managers can become more "cost conscious" in the care planning process.

Major Loss or Crisis

Another targeting criterion involved whether the client had experienced a major loss or crisis, such as the death of spouse or loss of long-term residence. Under this criterion, concern is for the possible harmful effect that such a change can have on a frail older person's life. In Project OPEN, the loss could have occurred within the preceding 12 months. MSSP guidelines simply indicated that the loss must have occurred "recently."

Unmet Needs/Fragile Informal Support System

The "unmet needs" criterion was used in the Channeling Demonstration to identify individuals needing help in at least two categories as a result of changes in functional impairment that occurred within the previous six months (including assistance with meals, housework/ shopping, medications, medical treatments at home, and personal care). Unmet needs could be present because clients did not have access to available services, or because services did not exist in their community.

In Channeling Demonstration criteria, it was possible to substitute the presence of "fragile informal support system" for the unmet needs criterion. Using this criterion, it was possible to identify clients whose caregivers were reaching the point of "burnout," or were ill themselves and would not have been able to care for the client. Using this targeting criterion might serve a preventive function by anticipating a situation in which client and caregiver needs for formally provided services could increase if the family is not supported or given respite services.

Assessments of social and environmental factors, such as the status of a client's informal support system, have also been conducted to determine the risk of institutionalization. In a review of 26 states' applications for Medicaid 2176 waivers, one study noted that while 70 percent of the states collected this "nonmedical" information, only 37 percent used it in making level-of-care decisions (Greenberg, Schmitz, & Lakin, 1983).

GATEKEEPING

Gatekeeping mechanisms are designed to control the number and types of services that clients receive, particularly high cost services such as institutional care. The gatekeeping mechanisms addressed in this section are interrelated, but have been separated for analytic and discussion purposes. Targeting and gatekeeping are closely related; effective and efficient targeting influences the kinds of gatekeeping mechanisms that are in place in a given delivery system. Both targeting and gatekeeping can affect the costs of long-term care service delivery.

Authorization Power and Purchase Capacity

A case manager's power to purchase services is determined by the range of services that can be authorized, the availability of these services in the local delivery system, and the designation of the case manager as the fiscally accountable person. Case managers with authorization power (as in Channeling, South Carolina, 2176, S/HMO) are fiscally accountable for the care plans they develop. Costs of individual client care plans are usually limited by the specified cap in an individual program. Care plans may also be subject to agency or caseload budget caps.

While case managers in the Financial Control model of Channeling and other long-term care demonstration projects could authorize an extensive list of community-based services, their authorization power did not extend to hospital, nursing home, or physician care. Physicians maintained the authority to make decisions in these areas. A case manager's power to prescribe and order services is also influenced by other factors such as the supply of community-based services in the local delivery system, and negotiated unit costs for various services.

Cap on Expenditures

A specific budgetary control mechanism used by some case management demonstrations and programs involved setting a maximum amount or "cap" on average expenditures for the program's entire caseload. For example, in the Financial Control Channeling sites, expenditures for the entire caseload were limited to 60 percent of the costs of nursing home care. Under this system, care plans for individual clients could vary as long as the total project budget remained under the 60 percent cap. This provision allowed case managers to develop care plans that were higher than the average cost for some clients if these were balanced by other lower cost care plans (Carcagno, et al, 1986).

Other programs used a cost limit on individual client care plans, in addition to or instead of an overall caseload budget cap. States providing case management under the Medicaid 2176 waiver program can choose to automatically deny services if a client's initial care plan indicates that the cost of community care will exceed the specified percentage of the cost of institutional care. Forty-six percent of the initial states providing services to the aged under the 2176 waiver incorporated this cost containment feature (Greenberg, et al., 1983). Other states may choose not to deny community services to clients whose initial care plans exceed the budget cap in situations, for example, when provision of community-based care is high initially, but expected to decrease as the client's situation stabilizes over time.

The Channeling Demonstration set a maximum individual client expenditure cap at 85 percent of the cost of state nursing home care. State approval was required for any client whose care plan exceeded that limit. Individuals whose care plan exceeded the cap could be served as long as these costs were offset by other clients whose care plans fell below the cost cap.

New York's Nursing Home Without Walls program operated under an individual client cap at 75 percent of the state ICF and SNF rates. This program's care plan costs included all home health services and treatments received by clients whether or not those services were coordinated by the program. The individual budget cap was calculated on an annual basis, providing case managers with enough flexibility to go above the cap during some months as long as the client care plan dipped below the cap in other months and averaged out to 75 percent for the year. This provision enabled large one-time expenses to be prorated over a number of months. Such expenses included architectural modifications to the client's home and/or purchase of major medical equipment.

The family budget cap is an interesting recommendation that emerged from experience gained in the New York Nursing Home Without Walls Program. It is used in situations where more than one client in a household needs the services of the program. Pooling individual budgets increased flexibility, and in some cases helped to keep clients together and in the community for longer than would otherwise be possible (Kodner, Mossey, & Dapello, 1984).

A variation on the concept of individual client budget caps was used in the Ukiah, California site of the MSSP project. Client expenditures were determined by assignment to one of three "risk categories." Clients were assigned to a category depending on their assessed risk of being institutionalized. The cost limits of each category represented a percentage of the comparable cost of nursing home care (e.g., 100%, 70%, and 55%). After categorizing each, case managers reviewed costs on a monthly basis to identify clients who were exceeding or falling below their assigned cost category.

Coale (1983) noted that this individual client cost limitation system was useful to clients and their families when a client reached his or her expenditure ceiling and additional planning was required. These limitations provided a "convenient peg for clients to hang difficult decisions on" (Coale, 1983). In these situations families may decide to increase their efforts in caring for their relative, clients may choose to do without certain services in order to remain at home, or the need to move into a nursing home may become apparent. The structure provided by the cost limit categories helped put these difficult decisions in perspective and assured clients and families that all alternative care plans had been fully explored.

Provider Risk

Provider risk is a central feature of the Social/HMO, On Lok, and other prospectively reimbursed systems. Provider risk is increased when financial responsibility and liability for long-term care expenditures are shifted to provider organizations. Provider organizations can remain financially afloat within a prospective payment system if they keep costs below the predetermined aggregate capitation rate. The provider organization is then at financial risk for expenses exceeding the prepaid amount. Leutz et al. (1985) identified three rationales for increasing provider risk through prepayment. This approach is designed to: enhance efficiency; link fiscal accountability to capacity to control costs; and increase capacity to predict the dynamics of revenues, expenditures, and budgeting. Provider risk creates incentives for providers to control total costs, to provide and promote preventive health care practices, and to substitute lower cost community-based services for higher cost hospital and nursing home care where appropriate.

Centralized Authorization Power

Centralization of authority to allocate resources is the degree to which case managers have discretion to use a broad scope of resources and related funding. The maximum degree of centralized authority is found in programs where a case manager authorizes, funds, and terminates a wide range of services for her or his clients, including acute and ambulatory health care. Currently, this broad authorization power is seen only in consolidated model programs like the Social/HMO and On Lok. The consolidated model (Leutz et al 1985) incorporates the following characteristics: a comprehensive array of health and social services are provided through a single program; care planners and service providers work closely and in some cases are one and the same; there is an enhanced capacity to exert fiscal control through management of all service expenditures. In the Social/HMO, the total range of services is made available to enrollees through one administrative structure (Leutz, et al., 1985). The single provider is responsible for both acute and long-term care needs of its members in the community and/or in institutions. This integration is designed to provide easier access to appropriate services by eliminating artificial barriers between medical and social support services. Case management authority in the Social/HMO project sites is potentially great, depending on the working relationships case managers develop with project site physicians.

The On Lok demonstration has evolved through several stages. At its inception, On Lok was designed to provide day health services to the elderly of the Chinatown and North Beach-Polk areas of San Francisco. Beginning in 1983, On Lok shifted its funding from sole reliance on Medicare to incorporation of traditional long-term care payment sources (Medicaid, private insurance, co-payments, and Medicare). Medicare waivers permitted prospective payment of a capitation rate rather than payment based on service unit costs. Zawadski and Ansak (1984) have stated that the ultimate objective of On Lok as a consolidated system has been the assumption of risk. Control over the generation of costs through care planning has been enhanced in On Lok since most services are provided directly by On Lok staff, many of whom are involved in the initial intake and assessment process. The intake and assessment teams function collectively as clients' case managers. On Lok has centralized several case management tasks (intake, assessment, care planning, monitoring, and reassessment) in the intake and assessment team, which also directly provides services to clients.

Financial Control Channeling was another example of centralized case manager authority, although the authority was not as broad as in the Social/HMO or On Lok. In this project, funding from Medicare, Medicaid, Title III of the Older Americans Act, and Social Services Block Grant (Title XX) was pooled. Case managers could authorize services using the funds pool without having to establish client eligibility for each program. This authority did not, however, extend to acute, ambulatory, and institutional care plan decisionmaking.

The amount of discretion a case manager has over funding allocation is central to his or her capacity to affect provider behavior. Austin (1983) has suggested that a centralized case management system, especially one with a single point of entry, can minimize the ability of service providers to resist case manager decisions (Austin, 1983).

Case managers' capacity to contain service costs is largely dependent upon the kind and amount of gatekeeping authority they have. Gatekeeping authority also affects a case manager's ability to act as a change agent in the local delivery system. With authority comes accountability, as well as increased case manager awareness of the costs and effects of the services they authorize. The potential of case managers to contain long-term care costs through their gatekeeping activities needs further examination. The case manager role is becoming more complex, including several key components such as management, advocacy, monitoring, gatekeeping, and concern for clients' and caregivers' welfare.

ORGANIZATIONAL AUSPICES

Case management can be delivered from a variety of organizational settings: service providing agencies, independent case management organizations, Area Agencies on Aging, and hospitals. Case management can also be provided from a variety of bureaucratic/geographic levels: state, regional, and local.

To date, there is no clear evidence suggesting the best organizational location for effective case management. There are trade-offs associated with each choice. In making these decisions, several issues should be examined, including the community's long-term care delivery system, and organizational and staff capacity. It is important to realize that the case management role and how it is performed will be directly influenced by the organizational setting. The following discussion examines alternative approaches to various levels and organizational locations from which case management can be delivered.

Location of Case Management by Level in a Service Delivery System

State Level. When a case management program is administered from a state level agency, with case managers located in the communities, the program can be more systematically designed and implemented throughout the state. A state level location also enhances the potential to facilitate coordination among multiple state agencies involved in long-term care. MSSP is an example of a state administered case management system.

MSSP is sponsored by the California State Health and Welfare Agency, and has its central administrative office in that agency. Case management is provided in local sites located throughout the state. As a state sponsored project, MSSP has strong system-level goals. These goals include: 1) reducing public expenditures for health and social services; 2) coordinating the long-term care delivery system; 3) filling service gaps in the continuum of care; and 4) testing a model of care that may provide a basis for a future statewide delivery system (Capitman, et al., 1983).

Area Level. The "service area" or regional location for case management activities is exemplified by the Area Agencies on Aging (AAAs). In its "Community-Based Long-Term Care Statement," the National Association of Area Agencies on Aging (N4A) recommended that Area Agencies on Aging be mandated, through changes in the Older Americans Act, to have the primary responsibility for developing case management systems in their areas and for coordinating federal and state funds for services to the elderly (National Association of Area Agencies, 1984). Language added to the 1984 Older Americans Act created new case management responsibilities for the AAAs:

> to conduct efforts to facilitate the coordination of community-based long-term care services designed to retain individuals in their homes thereby deferring unnecessary, costly institutionalization, and designed to emphasize the development of client centered case management systems as a component of such services (Older Americans Act, 1984).

The National Association of Area Agencies on Aging argued that AAA involvement in case management has evolved "in a grass roots fashion" in response to specific needs in different communities (National Association of Area Agencies on Aging, 1984). The N4A asserted that responsibility for providing community-based long-term care systems needs to be at the local level, with management and planning occurring in an autonomous, nonprovider agency that has service area jurisdiction. Several State Units on Aging (SUAs) and AAAs have been successful in promoting this approach and have developed effective community-based long-term care systems in a number of communities.

For example, Arkansas and Florida have been successful in developing and coordinating long-term care delivery systems in their states at the AAA level. AAAs in Arkansas are Medicaid certified and provide case management services for Medicaid-eligible clients as well as for private paying clients. Two of the eight AAAs in Arkansas function as gatekeepers for nursing home admission. These agencies do not, however, provide direct services.

AAAs in Florida administer the statewide Community Care for the Elderly (CCE) system for functionally impaired older persons. The program helps functionally impaired older persons remain in the least restrictive environment suitable to their needs. The AAAs designate lead agencies to: provide case management or assure its provision; provide or subcontract for community-based services; compile community care statistics; and monitor provider agencies under contract with the AAAs [(N4A)—Models of community-based long-term care systems, n.d.]

Local Level. A case management agency that operates from the local level is more likely to be perceived as part of the local delivery system. Case managers may be in a better position to form partnerships with providers by using this approach. The increased proximity may help case managers to foster greater coordination among agencies. The Long-Term Care Project of North San Diego County is an example of a local level project. The project was located in a local home health care agency, Allied Home Health Associates (AHHA). Its single site served about 10% of the elders in need of services in its catchment area. AHHA contracted for services with 18 other providers, including two other home health agencies (Capitman, 1983).

A possible disadvantage of this approach is that providers may perceive competition between themselves and the case management agency. Friction can result if providers attempt to "sabotage" the case management effort in their community by withholding appropriate referrals and resisting efforts to eliminate duplications in assessment and monitoring activities.

Mixed. The state of Oregon utilizes a mixed system. Oregon's Senior Services Division (SSD) is the only fully integrated state-level long-term care agency in the nation. At the service area level, AAAs at their own choice can implement local case management systems.

These Type "B" AAAs have the authority to manage all long-term care funds, including Medicaid, Social Services Block Grant, and Oregon Project Independence. They also operate the nursing home pre-admission screening program and coordinate local systems of long-term care.

Other individual AAAs in the state of Oregon have chosen not to assume this authority. In these Type "A" AAAs, staff administer the Older American Act programs and Oregon Project Independence funds (state general funds), while the State administers Medicaid and Social Service Block Grant programs. In these cases, case management is provided from the state SSD office.

Currently 13 of the 18 AAAs in Oregon have chosen the Type "B" option. Type "B" AAAs are required to collect data, assess the needs of the population they serve, prepare long-range plans for their geographic area, and develop a comprehensive, coordinated system of care (e.g., through case management). Area agencies vary in terms of their capacity to manage the kind of complex programs administered by the Type "B" Area Agencies in Oregon. Allowing individual AAAs to decide whether to accept expanded authority and responsibility recognizes these differences. Some area agencies are more able to handle this expanded role and responsibility than others.

Location of Case Management by Type of Organization

Like organizational auspices, it is not clear that one organizational location for case management is superior to another. Table 3–5 provides a comparative assessment of the advantages and disadvantages of locating case management in five kinds of organizations. The following discussion highlights key issues related to this decision.

Freestanding Agency. Locating case management in a freestanding agency provides a measure of autonomy and may avoid conflict of interest problems that can arise when case management and direct services are offered by the same agency. Case managers employed by a disinterested freestanding agency are not pressured to incorporate their own agency's services into care plans. If the freestanding agency can establish credibility within the local delivery system and overcome the hurdle of provider resistance to case manager control, the autonomous, disinterested organization can be an advantageous location. If the program gives case managers the authority to purchase services for its clients, such care planning decisions will directly affect the local service delivery system through the distribution of resources. Armed with this authority, case managers can reward efficient providers with referrals and contracts.

If a new freestanding agency is created, however, the advantages could be outweighed by the problems associated with start up difficulties encountered in developing a new local organization. In this situation, several problems can be anticipated, including: 1) front-end costs, e.g., expenses associated with starting a new organization from the ground up such as purchasing supplies, equipment, and renting space; 2) time and investment needed for program planning and public relations, e.g., staff salaries and benefits paid prior to when clients begin to be served, designing, planning, and advertising the program to the community; 3) total responsibility for overhead, e.g., r ⁓⁓ipment, furniture, and utilities; 4) maintenance costs, e.g., (⁓⁓air of office and equipment, and 5) establishing an ⁓ the total delivery system, e.g., the time it ' accepted by the local providers and

⁓ning agencies such as AAAs
` management. This loca-
'ent case management
⁓dgeable about and
⁓ts are frequently
⁓ncy staff may be
aᴠᴌe to provide consultation and facilitate pᵣᴠ⁓ ⁓m-solving in planning for the provision of services.

The National Association of Area Agencies on Aging has suggested that responsibility for long-term care case management be vested in AAAs or their designated contractors (National Association of Area Agencies on Aging, 1984). Their advocacy mandate may mean that the AAAs have visibility in their local communities, and their planning responsibility may mean that they are likely to have working relationships with many community providers. All AAAs are not presently capable of performing case management. Many, however, could assume this role with appropriate preparation and time for capacity building.

Special Unit in an Information and Referral Agency. Another possible location for case management is as a unit within a centralized information and referral (I & R) agency. A case management program could be set up as a separate unit and could receive referrals directly from I & R workers. Clients who contact the I & R agency for assistance could be screened to determine if they need case management based on its targeting criteria, e.g., need a comprehensive assessment, multiple services, and monitoring. These potential clients could be referred directly to case managers with preliminary

TABLE 3–5 Organization Auspices for Case Management Programs

1. Freestanding agency

Advantages	Disadvantages
autonomy free of historical organizational policies & practices avoids conflict of interest with internal direct service provision fewer constraints in making program modifications (can be helpful in securing new funding)	local credibility can be difficult to establish more subject to case flow problems (as a single-purpose agency is more vulnerable to rise and fall of funding) start up problems provider resistance

2. Special unit in a planning agency
(e.g., Area Agency on Aging or public social services department)

Advantages	Disadvantages
more visible, easier for clients to locate more influence with service providers who seek funds enhanced access to clients, funds, and special expertise potential for administrative costs to be subsumed by larger organization close access to program planners who may assist in filling service gaps and responding to deficiencies in quality of services.	planning agency administrator's concerns may be more interorganizational and political than client-oriented conflicts planning agency may have with service providers could spill over and affect case managers' relationships with clients

3. Special unit in an I & R agency

Advantages	Disadvantages
established referral resources viewed as nonthreatening and noncompetitive by the local providers its image is not stereotyped in terms of types of client or services staff are experienced in screening and referral awareness of existing gaps in community services	history of inadequate funding and inability to afford competent personnel can result in negative reputations associated with some I & R agencies

TABLE 3–5 (Continued)

4. Special unit in a provider agency	
Advantages	Disadvantages
some providers have accumulated experience in working with homebound elderly some already have or can readily recruit case managers existing policies, personnel, and case-finding techniques can be compatible with case management program	potential conflict of interest in assessing need and purchasing services

5. Special unit in a hospital	
Advantages	Disadvantages
potential benefit from nonstigmatized reputation of hospital advantageous location for case-finding frail elderly advantageous location for diverting people from nursing home opportunity to educate physicians about alternatives to nursing home care potentially solid funding basis opportunity for involvement in acute care planning on-site health care professionals available for consultations and special assessments	potentially difficult to gain acceptance within the larger hospital potentially difficult to gain extra resources required for case management potential conflict with hospital discharge planners (need for clear role definition) potential difficulty in convincing hospital of need to continue monitoring clients in order to avoid unnecessary hospitalization

Adapted from Steinberg, R. and Carter, G. (1983). *Case Management and the Elderly.* Lexington, MA: Lexington Books.

paperwork completed by the I & R workers. Including case management in an I & R agency may represent a major change in orientation for the I & R organization. Although it may be difficult to locate an I & R agency that would be willing to incorporate a whole new unit, this approach has been implemented in the Senior Information and Assistance Program in Seattle, Washington (Austin, et al, 1985).

Special Unit in a Provider Agency. One of the key issues regarding location is whether placement within a provider agency could permit sufficient autonomy for case managers. The question is whether a case manager employed by a provider could maintain objectivity during assessment and care planning. There may be a conflict of interest for the provider-employed case manager. These case managers may feel pressured to identify needs that could be met by services provided by their own agency. On the other hand, provider agencies may have more intimate knowledge about clients, their histories, and needs. This familiarity could facilitate client acceptance of case management.

Whether a case management agency should also provide services depends on the kinds and amounts of resources available in the community, as well as the financial incentives faced by the agency. In a service-poor area, it may be neither efficient nor possible to work with independent providers. For example, many rural counties may have only a single provider of home or community-based care, e.g., the Visiting Nurses' Association or the county welfare department.

In terms of financial incentives, agencies operating with fixed budgets would have no incentive to overprescribe services. Under these conditions, agencies would provide their own services only if they could do it at a lower cost or with higher quality (Greenberg, Doth, & Austin, 1981). Therefore, combining service delivery and case management may be feasible. However, if such an approach were used, a mechanism to ensure the independence of case-management decision-making would be essential.

Special Unit in a Hospital. Hospitals are emerging as another possible location for case management, potentially enabling more effective targeting of frail elderly patients who may be inpatients, outpatients, or who have entered the hospital's emergency room. Hospital discharge is a critical time for determining if an elderly person needs nursing home care or could manage in the community with appropriate services. Hospital discharge may also result in temporary placement in a nursing home and subsequent discharge plans once rehabilitation has been completed. The hospital setting allows case managers to gain access to the skills and expertise of numerous health care professionals who may be available for consultation and special assessments.

A hospital-based case management program will necessarily include physicians, nurses, and other health care professionals who may claim authority for resource allocation and expect participation in care plan decision-making. On the other hand, given DRG discharge pressure, case managers may assist hospital staff with assessment, facilitate discharge, and provide an important link to community providers. Case managers can educate physicians about community-based services that may prevent unnecessary nursing home placements.

The Robert Wood Johnson Foundation has stimulated the development of hospital-based long-term care programs through its "Hospital Initiatives in Long-Term Care" program. The Foundation has funded 24 hospitals to plan, develop, and implement new roles for hospitals in their communities' long-term care delivery systems. Case management and the integration of long-term care with traditional hospital services are common features of these projects. Funding for these projects terminated in 1988. Evaluation findings indicate substantial variation among the hospitals in case management models, staffing, and target populations (Capitman, et.al., 1988).

Chapter 4

Case Management Design Options

Any specific case management program can vary along a number of dimensions, each of which can affect both program effectiveness and client outcomes. Some of this variation can be traced to choices made in the process of designing the program, some may be dictated by the statutory authority of the case management agency, and some of the variation may be a function of the local service delivery environment. In this section, drawing upon the operational experience of the major long-term care demonstrations, the key program options that must be considered in designing a case managed system are discussed. Key design options include:

interface with the local delivery system

case manager's tasks and functions

case management staffing and levels of professionalization

individual vs. team approach

case manager authority

case manager interface with the health care system

timing of the case management intervention

caseload size and mix

intensity of the case manager-client relationship

Developing case management services requires exploration of these major design issues.

LOCAL DELIVERY SYSTEM

The relationship between the organizational auspices of the case management program and the character of the community's service delivery system requires careful analysis. Two issues are addressed: 1) single versus multiple agency involvement in case management; and 2) the extent to which various case management functions are split among different agencies. The environment of the local delivery system must be taken into consideration when exploring the alternatives.

Since delivery systems and their capacities vary so much from one community to another, it is unlikely that a single choice for locating a case management program will work in every location. To comprehensively assess the local delivery system, program planners must examine: 1) system comprehensiveness (how complete is the continuum of care?); 2) its bias toward institutional care; 3) its complexity (how dense is the population of providers; how many duplications, overlaps, and gaps exist?); and 4) its quality. A comprehensive listing of delivery system contextual variables is provided in Table 4–1. Case management program planning includes an analysis and examination of the dynamics within the local delivery system that will influence the choice of organizational auspices for the case management program. Further, it will be necessary to determine providers' power to thwart case managers' authority.

> A more centralized case management system with a single point of entry would minimize the power of service providers to resist case management controls. Because providers can be expected to try to protect whatever power they possess in dealing with case managers, level of centralization is a key issue (Austin, 1983, p. 25).

Following an analysis of the local delivery system, any agency considering the development of a case management program must also thoroughly examine its own characteristics. Table 4–2 summarizes the categories and types of information that should be included in an agency profile. Specification of client characteristics is critical to understanding the potential market for case management services among the agency's current clients. This analysis will also provide valuable information regarding other possible client populations the agency might want to target for case management services.

Although agency staff may believe they fully understand and ap-

TABLE 4–1 Case Management Service Delivery Context

Perceptions and relationships	Facilities and services available
• Historical character of relationships among actors • Character of working relationships among agencies • Referral patterns • Degree of domain consensus • Nature of attitudes about other agencies • Identification of powerful actors • Assessment of system components open to manipulation • Local capacity for service expansion • Local capacity for innovation The community • Demographics • Age • Income • Living arrangements • Occupations The controls • Local • State • National • Specialty colleges (e.g., American College of Surgeons Cancer Center Program) • Joint Commission on Accreditation of Health Care Organizations (JCAHO) • Other accrediting agencies • Insurance companies • Zoning	Nursing homes • Ratio of beds to population 65+ • Ratio of SNF to ICF beds • Occupancy rates • Major referral patterns • Admissions and discharge patterns • Case mix • Reimbursement rates Hospitals • Utilization rates for population 65+ • Occupancy rates • Nature of discharge planning • Home care services available • Referral patterns Community health and social service agencies • Types of agencies • Number of agencies • Services provided • Number of people 65+ served • Service utilization patterns • Referral patterns • Cost per unit of service • Major funding sources • Short run service expansion capacity • Case management activities The competition • How many and who are they? • Services • Location • Occupancy • Medical staff • Programs • Affiliations • Future plans

preciate their agency's culture, mission, and operating preferences, a comprehensive review of agency characteristics is necessary to determine whether a case management program would be consistent with agency goals. Sources of support and resistance should be identified, so that potential implementation barriers can be anticipated. Percep-

TABLE 4–2 Agency Profile

Clients
  Age
  Sex
  Marital status
  Housing status
  Health status
  Income
  Length of association with agency
  Services used
  Use of other community services

The organization
  Mission
  Personnel
  Services
  Location
  Corporate structure
  Board composition
  Reputation
  Image
  Affiliations
  Outreach programs
  Educational activities

Agency staff
  Experience
  Specialty-credentials
  Time availability for new programs

tions and preferences of agency staff are critical to successful initiation and implementation of any new program. Case management program planners need a thorough understanding of how staff support can be marshalled and the extent to which current agency staff possess knowledge and skills necessary for the new program. Only after a comprehensive analysis of the agency's external delivery system context and a thorough examination of its internal environment is it possible to address other organizational auspices issues. Several of these issues are addressed below.

Depending on its statutory authority, a case management agency may be designated as the single point of entry into the community's long-term care delivery system. This agency could be responsible for all case management tasks. Whether one agency is capable of performing all case management tasks for an entire community, or if, instead, the responsibility should be shared with other agencies, depends on the individual community and its unique characteristics.

It is of primary importance that a case management program be implemented as a local operation, and on a small enough scale so that relationships can be developed with service providers. As Sterthous (1983) pointed out, just how "local should local be" depends upon the geographic size of the service area, the population density, and agency market share in each area.

Decisions about whether a case management agency should perform all or some case management functions must also be considered in light of local delivery system dynamics. Political advantages may be gained by contracting for parts of the case management function with existing community agencies. This strategy may enhance service coordination among community providers.

There are, however, potential problems inherent in involving providers in case management. To the extent that providers are involved in assessment and care planning, the potential exists for conflict of interest. For example, client assessment for appropriateness for community-based care is an important activity in which providers could conceivably play a major role. In a review of provider involvement in the assessment and case management functions in state programs developed under the Medicaid 2176 waiver authority, researchers found that, in 50 percent of these programs, providers developed the plan of care (Greenberg, et al., 1983).

Financial incentives could affect provider judgment in care plan development. In addition, while there has been considerable rhetoric about supporting rather than supplanting clients' informal support systems through the provision of formal services, it may be difficult for providers to embrace this goal given their own self-interest. This potential conflict of interest could result in higher than necessary service costs. On the other hand, providers may be the most knowledgeable about the clients' situations and may be best qualified to make client care decisions. Potential conflict of interest may be minimized if the provider/case manager is only allowed to carry out care plans designed by others.

Whether case management functions should be carried out in a local service area by one or more organizations or levels of government is an important management issue. While the system may be more efficient if one organization is responsible for all functions, this efficiency may not outweigh the cost of sacrificing important checks and balances.

The number of organizations or levels of government involved in providing case management or the ways in which those functions are distributed among community agencies may affect how the case management program interacts with other organizations in its local delivery system. More likely, case management's influence in its community's long-term care delivery system will be based on both its statutory authority and its ability to provide incentives and sanctions to providers. Further, in the future, it is likely that the quality of case management service delivery will become an increasingly significant selection criteria regarding organizational auspices for the service. Increased attention to quality assurance, standards for case managers' training, and demands for increased reliability in assessment and care planning will significantly influence the location of case management programs.

CASE MANAGER'S TASKS AND FUNCTIONS

Tasks and functions emerge differently as increasing authority is introduced into the case manager role. They are also influenced by the program context.

As authority increases for gatekeeping in terms of controlling access to services and budgetary constraints, the care planning process takes on added significance. Case managers operating under client and/or agency budget caps on care plans are fiscally accountable for the plans they develop. In six long-term care demonstration projects, case managers developed care plans with client budget caps (South Carolina Community Long-Term Care Project, ACCESS, Oregon's FIG/Waiver, MSSP, Georgia's AHS, and Channeling). As case managers have increased fiscal authority and responsibility for care planning, they function as resource allocators.

The local delivery system in which case managers operate also influences case management tasks and functions. The ACCESS project was implemented in Monroe County, New York, a county in which the continuum of community-based care is more completely developed compared to other communities around the state. Case managers working in this kind of a "service rich" environment (i.e., where many services are available, both in terms of number and type) may spend considerable time and effort in selecting, negotiating, and arranging services with providers. Case managers who can authorize, purchase, and terminate services for their clients may also have responsibility to monitor providers. Selecting providers and monitoring service delivery in a service rich community represent complex case management tasks.

On the other hand, case managers working in a "service poor" area, perhaps a rural community, may have comparatively few choices in performing these tasks. Case managers working in a "service poor" delivery system have the primary task of enhancing client access to the limited number of services that are available. In such communities, case managers may also engage in program development activities.

The population targeted for the program also affects case managers' responsibilities. Some case management programs are tied to a preadmission screening process and target clients who are about to enter nursing homes. In these programs, care planning includes authorization of locus (home or community) and level (ICF/SNF) of care. In contrast, other programs target community residents who are not at immediate risk of institutionalization. In these programs, level of care decisions are not a part of the case management function.

STAFFING AND LEVELS OF PROFESSIONALIZATION

Differing opinions exist over the levels and types of professional background needed to perform various case management functions. Case management staff in the Long-Term Care Demonstration Projects were, for the most part, professionally trained individuals, usually master's level social workers and/or registered nurses (Haskins et al., 1985; Kemper et al., 1987). In these projects, paraprofessionals (i.e., nondegree, associate degree, or bachelor's level workers) tended to screen, arrange, and monitor services. A recent study of case managers employed in public programs in Washington and Oregon reported that equal numbers of case managers believed that a bachelor's degree or less should be required for case managers. Only 8.5 percent of the respondents thought a master's degree was appropriate (Institute on Aging, University of Washington 1987).

Sterthous (1983) reviewed staffing patterns in 14 case management agencies. Only three of these agencies used paraprofessionals in the primary case management tasks of assessment, care planning, and service arrangement. The reasons given for using paraprofessional case management staff included: local norms favoring the use of paraprofessionals; a feeling that paraprofessionals were perceived as less of a threat by clients; cost factors; and beliefs that professionals tended to be too clinically oriented. Sterthous reported that professional case managers were used in each of the remaining projects. The primary reason for using professionals was the belief that case management was considered a skilled task, despite the use of a objective assessment tool. A leap needs to be made from information gathering (assessment) to decision-making (care planning). This is viewed as an extremely delicate and difficult process. (Sterthous, 1983).

In this same study, Sterthous compared the tasks performed by staff in projects using professionally trained case managers to those using paraprofessionals, and found no differences. The use of professional or paraprofessional case managers was influenced by the relative sophistication or comprehensiveness of the service system in which the case manager operated. Where fewer services were available, or where the case manager's authority was limited, less judgment was required, and therefore less professional training and experience was assumed to be needed. Others have argued that in this environment, case managers actually need a higher level of skill. The amount of supervision available and the opportunity for on-the-job training also influenced the level of professionalization. Closer supervision and training permitted hiring staff with less professional background, resulting in cost savings for the program.

INDIVIDUAL VS. TEAM APPROACH

Whether case management should be performed by one individual or a team is another unresolved issue. In several programs, teams are used for assessment and care planning in order to obtain a balance of professional input (psycho/social and medical) and to comprehensively address all aspects of a client's needs. Many of the demonstrations used teams for care planning while others used teams only for assessment.

Grisham and White (1982) examined the use of teams in case management, and summarized the advantages and disadvantages of the team approach. They identified the following advantages: 1) broader perspective; 2) peer support; and 3) shared decision-making. Team conflict is a potential danger, as is the possibility that no one individual is ultimately responsible and, therefore, services are ineffective. A survey of 93% of the MSSP case management staff, however, revealed strong support and enthusiasm for the team approach (Grisham and White, 1982). Often a social worker and a registered nurse work together as a team for assessment and care planning purposes. Potential for conflict exists here due in part to disagreement about which profession has the most relevant expertise (Amerman, 1983).

Another difficult issue is the cost associated with the participation of several highly paid professionals on teams. Group decisionmaking can be a waste of time and money, especially in the development of care plans. Involving too many expensive professionals may simply cost more, without added benefit to the clients. Professional input can be gained through consultations and special assessments, thereby limiting costly professional staff involvement in routine team activities. This modified team approach can also include peer supervision and external care plan review.

AUTHORITY

If care planning is viewed as a resource allocation activity, the kind and amount of authority case managers have to purchase services is an important program design variable. The Channeling demonstration is perhaps the clearest example of this key element. This demonstration project included two models, basic and financial control. Case managers in the five basic Channeling sites functioned primarily as brokers in their local service systems. Standardized care planning included recording client problems, anticipated outcomes, types of service needed, providers to be involved, and service delivery schedules. At the financial control sites, case managers also completed a cost worksheet that projected the costs of each service and of the entire care plan. However, they could independently order services for their clients. Since financial control case managers could directly purchase services, they decided on how much service to buy, times and days of service provision, and whether to terminate services or change the provider agency. There was only a limited amount of provider input. By contrast, case managers at the basic sites, who could not directly purchase services, had to negotiate their service requests with providers. These case managers found that their requests might be modified or denied; they sometimes encountered long delays before response. Negotiation was the primary method by which basic Channeling case managers implemented their care plans (Carcagno, et al., 1986).

Austin (1983) specified three core elements of case manager's authority: span of authority, scope of authority, and financial incentives. Span of authority refers to the extent of the case manager's access to or control over funding. Case managers operating with the widest span of authority control allocation of all funds available to members of a specific population from a variety of different sources (for example, Medicaid, Medicare, Social Services Block Grant, Title III of the Older Americans' Act).

Scope of authority refers to what case managers can do with the funds they control. Case managers operating with a broad scope control funds for prior authorization, preadmission screening, discharge planning, and follow-up with clients admitted to nursing homes. Case managers with a narrow scope of authority only control funds to monitor the development of service plans and contracts with providers.

Case management can be designed to include financial incentives and sanctions. Such incentives might be used to develop services missing in the local continuum of care. Sanctions can also serve as cost control measures, for example, target budgets for individual agencies and clients, ceilings on budgets of specific catchment areas, and capitation of funding.

CASE MANAGER INTERFACE WITH THE HEALTH CARE SYSTEM

While the importance of nonmedical factors in assessing need and appropriateness for long-term care services is broadly acknowledged,

> physicians as gatekeepers have tended to consider social and environmental factors (isolation, lack of any familial or other informal supports, difficulties or inadequacies of living arrangements, need for transportation, counseling, supervision, etc.) beyond their concerns, time consuming, and outside their professional preparation (Simpson, 1982, p. 64).

Quality long-term care planning requires a balance between psycho/ social and medical perspectives. Case managers can be in a position to develop and maintain this balance.

Physicians are concerned about the fact that they are ultimately responsible for the care of their patients and are potentially liable for malpractice. Until liability is shared by case management agencies, physicians cannot surrender their authority (Grisham & White, 1982). Routinely involving physicians in the assessment and care planning process must be weighed against the high cost of physician time. Geriatric medical assessment can identify treatable conditions that may alter clients' functional capacities. The presence of a medical director and access to medical consultation are two possible strategies.

Reviewing the long-term care demonstrations indicates that physicians have not been actively involved in the case management process in these projects. In two studies, physicians had no formal role. In two other projects (San Diego and New York's Home Care Project), physicians were only occasionally involved, primarily as members of the care planning team. Physician involvement in four of the demonstrations (Triage, South Carolina Community Long-Term Care, and Channeling) took the form of case managers regularly communicating with each client's physician.

Three of the long-term care projects used physicians on a regular basis. On Lok staff physicians were part of the care planning team and were involved in all other aspects of case management. Florida's Pentastar project contracted for physician services for assessment and care planning. Project OPEN at Mount Zion Hospital attempted to involve clients' personal physicians in the care planning team, but had limited success. OPEN's staff cited problems with case management team care planning meetings interfering with physician office hours, physician confusion over OPEN's purpose, and concern over authority. As a substitute, postgraduate Fellows in Geriatric Medicine at Mount Zion Hospital became involved in team care planning, thus benefiting both the Fellows and Project OPEN.

Physicians have been most frequently involved in care planning. This is not surprising given the fact that they have historically been the traditional gatekeepers of long-term care resources. Medicaid certification for ICF or SNF levels of nursing home care and Medicaid and Medicare coverage of in-home medical care requires physician approval. Further, families frequently turn to physicians for advice on whether to move their elderly relative into a nursing home. In three projects, physician approval of client care plans was required: MSSP, Florida's Pentastar Project, and New York's Nursing Home Without Walls. It is not clear, however, whether this involvement was more than a paper review or telephone consultation.

TIMING OF THE CASE MANAGEMENT INTERVENTION

The point in time at which a client or client's family makes contact with a case manager can vary depending on program eligibility or targeting guidelines as well as individual client characteristics. Contact with a case manager may first occur when an elderly person applies for nursing home admission. If there is a preadmission screening (PAS) program in the state, the individual may be required to be assessed by a PAS team. If it is feasible for the patient to continue residing in the community, a care plan is developed and a case manager assigned. In Oregon, persons who are admitted to nursing homes are also assigned to a case manager who works with the client toward discharge, if feasible.

Some programs (e.g., North San Diego Long-Term Care Project, MSSP, Robert Wood Johnson Hospital in Initiatives in Long-Term Care Sites) target clients who are being discharged from hospitals or nursing homes after an acute illness. In this situation, the case manager is involved as part of the discharge planning process, and care planning focuses on in-home services that facilitate rehabilitation and convalescence at home. Case management involvement in these cases is triggered by an acute illness and subsequent discharge planning activities.

The timing of case manager involvement is difficult to specify when the client is not acutely ill and is residing in the community. Here the definition of client "spell of illness" becomes more vague. The question actually becomes: What is the precipitating event that triggers case manager involvement? One trigger is the "burn out" experienced by the spouse or other family members who have been providing care to the client and need assistance with caregiving (Carcagno, et al., 1986). The Channeling Project defined several other events in clients' lives that triggered reassessments, bringing clients and/or their caregivers into contact with case managers. Those events included: loss of a major caretaker through death or a move; death of a client's spouse or member of the household; acute medical crisis; major deterioration in physical or mental status; placement in a hospital or nursing home (Schneider & Weiss, 1982).

CASELOAD SIZE AND MIX

Caseload size is affected by a number of variables and reflects the agency's assumptions regarding the appropriate number of clients a case manager can handle. Caseload size is determined by a combination of factors such as the level of need for case management services existing in a community, eligibility requirements established for entry into the program, support for the case management program in the community, and the local availability of long-term care services.

Case mix is an important factor in determining caseload size. If the case manager is carrying a caseload of extremely frail clients, the number of cases a case manager can realistically handle is limited. In Channeling, there was very little case mix because almost all the clients experienced serious functional disability. In this situation, with caseloads of very impaired clients, 50 was recommended as a feasible number of clients for each case manager.

Caseload size in long-term care demonstration projects varied. For example, Florida's Pentastar had an average caseload size of 35 to 40; San Diego's Long-Term Care Project had a similar range, 37 to 46. MSSP's Senior Service Counselors (the most traditional case manager role in MSSP) carried caseloads of 50 to 67 clients. The caseload size of South Carolina's Community Long-Term Care Project was larger, averaging 75 to 85. This project also required a mandatory preadmission screening.

In a survey of MSSP case management staff, case managers were asked to specify an ideal caseload size (Grisham & White, 1982).

Respondents indicated that 30 to 50 clients represented an ideal number, although many indicated that this was probably unrealistic. MSSP case managers emphasized the importance of considering case mix when determining caseload size because working with some clients was more time consuming than others. In a time study, Grisham (1983) examined the issue of what constitutes a manageable caseload size for an entire caseload of clients on the threshold of institutionalization. The study explored how the intensity of case management varied by client characteristics in all eight of California's MSSP demonstration sites. The recommended caseload sizes were as follows: 58 for senior services counselors; 84 for health professionals; and 88 for senior service aides. Several factors were identified as significantly related to the intensity of case manager-client activities: 1) client movement from one residence to another; 2) clinical judgment of "threshold status" or client risk of institutionalization; and 3) caseload size. As caseload size increased, case managers reported a decreasing capability to perform "ongoing" case management activities such as follow-up, monitoring, and reassessment.

INTENSITY OF THE CASE MANAGER-CLIENT RELATIONSHIP

An issue that has received relatively little attention is the intensity of the relationship the case manager has with his or her clients. Amerman, Eisenberg, & Weisman (1983) reviewed case management practice literature and found that, although case management practice assumes a relationship exists between the case manager and the client, there is little description of what that interaction might be. Many case managers have training in social work or nursing. This educational background prepares nurses and social workers for the role of client advocate, acting on behalf of clients with the service providers, and the clients' informal support systems. Client counseling is sometimes a significant focus of case management activity. For example, 50 percent of MSSP's case managers stated that they counseled their clients. Although they acknowledged counseling was not in their job description, they recognized the need and provided the service (Grisham & White, 1982).

The trend in case management, however, has been toward a greater emphasis on gatekeeping. Case managers are being asked to more closely control access to scarce services. Some case managers are fiscally accountable for the costs of their clients' care plans such as those operating under client and/or agency budget caps. However, when the case manager is primarily a gatekeeper, with a large caseload, the nature of client relationships changes. In these situations, case managers are forced to rely primarily on reports from providers about the nature of clients' service needs and use this information in making care planning decisions. As a result, there actually may be no "relationship" between the case manager and the client.

The emphasis on cost consciousness for the case manager who is a gatekeeper of long-term care services appears to conflict with goals inherent in client advocacy or counseling. Client advocacy and counseling may not contribute to cost effective outcomes. It may be unrealistic to expect case managers to effectively carry out the responsibilities of both roles, although presently most programs include both advocacy and gatekeeping in their definitions of case management. A recent study in the northwest, however, indicated that case managers view their jobs as more complex, including five components of the role: managing, advocating, providing for clients'-caregivers' welfare, monitoring, and gatekeeping (University of Washington, Institute on Aging, 1987).

Without resolution of these conflicting goals, there cannot be a consensus on the nature of case manager-client relationships. If it is decided, in the interest of cost saving, that the appropriate role for the case manager is primarily that of gatekeeper, the question remains: Who, if anyone, has the client advocacy role? This is an important ethical issue affecting client choice and an issue deserving further consideration in the design of future long-term care programs and polices.

CLIENT OUTCOMES AND UTILIZATION COSTS

The long-term care demonstrations attempted to affect outcomes for clients by altering service utilization patterns. Attempts to measure client outcomes varied considerably across the studies, making an overall assessment of outcomes across projects difficult. Efforts to measure client life quality included several areas: unmet needs, satisfaction with service arrangements, social interaction, health and functioning, and longevity (Kemper, et al., 1987).

A review of results across these measures indicates that overall life quality was improved for program clients as a result of receiving expanded case-managed community services. Three projects (Channeling, Georgia, New York City Home Care) reported a reduction in unmet needs for program clients as compared to nonprogram clients. Two projects (Project OPEN and Basic Channeling) found significant increases in social interaction for program clients. Effects on functioning demonstrated somewhat mixed results, although the major finding was that functioning was not affected by program intervention. The life satisfaction of program clients was reported to be higher in each of the eight randomized research studies (Kemper, et.al., 1987), yet the size of the effects was generally small. Finally, in seven of the eight randomized studies, mortality was lower for program clients.

Outcomes in the area of cost and service utilization suggest that in most instances service utilization patterns were not altered to the extent expected. In general, those projects whose primary intervention strategy was designed to upgrade the package of home care services available in the community produced reductions in the use of hospital and nursing home care. These reductions, however, were offset by increases in the costs of waivered services and case management (Kemper et al., 1987). Studying the effects on cost is limited by the data collected and because comprehensive cost data are difficult to collect as they are dispersed across numerous providers and funding sources.

Two projects proved to be exceptions to these general findings that expanded community care resulted in overall increased costs. The South Carolina Community Long-Term Care Project, a preadmission screening program, directly diverted nursing home applicants, had lower use of traditional services, and essentially broke even on total costs. On Lok, the only consolidated model project BPA examined, reported cost savings, although that project had a limited research effort (Kemper, et al., 1987). Both projects targeted clients who were ICF and SNF certifiable. Results from the other long-term care demonstration projects indicate that, although total cost savings were not achieved, cost reduction was achieved for a subgroup of the most frail clients. These findings indicate that the ability to produce lower public costs in long-term care is directly associated with successfully targeting clients. Such targeting, however, appears difficult to implement, particularly without linking entry to a nursing home preadmission screening process.

The case management design options outlined in this chapter reflect the range of issues requiring attention by administrators and policymakers as they consider program development alternatives. These choices, however, are not made in a vacuum. The next chapter focuses on how design variables operationally affect case management service delivery.

Part **II**

EVALUATING AND ASSURING THE QUALITY OF CASE-MANAGED CARE

"Quite as important as legislation is vigilant oversight of administration" **WOODROW WILSON**

"Who shall guard the guardians themselves?" **JUVENAL**

"There are three kinds of lies: lies, damned lies, and statistics." **BENJAMIN DISRAELI** (1804–1881)

Chapter **5**

Evaluation and Quality Assurance of Case Management: An Overview

Despite the increase in the provision of case management and the completion of many research demonstrations, limited information has been available about how to *best monitor and evaluate the effectiveness* of case management. The following chapters present examples of different evaluative approaches and strategies used in recent community care demonstrations and in ongoing operating programs. This chapter will provide an overview of the monitoring and evaluation challenges faced by case management agencies. Chapter 6 will then examine quality assurance and monitoring strategies. Chapter 7 will then provide examples of evaluation efforts and issues.

WHY EVALUATE AND MONITOR CASE MANAGEMENT PROGRAMS?

Case management agencies must address the question of whether or not to monitor and evaluate program activities. Clearly, in some instances, agencies do not have a choice. However, agency personnel are often ambivalent about program evaluation. On the one hand, staff like to have information that can be used to demonstrate program effectiveness. On the other hand, they are often concerned about the costs and other potential difficulties associated with undertaking evaluative activities. Numerous barriers can deter agency action in undertaking program evaluation and quality assurance efforts. Common barriers include:

- An expectation that there will be an increase in the paperwork burden experienced by case managers who may already feel overwhelmed in this area
- Associating evaluation with a language that is often mostly jargon (such as two-tailed tests, internal reliability, Type 1 error), which is not part of the average practitioner's vocabulary
- The costliness of evaluation in terms of both staff time and agency dollars. Undertaking evaluation means making a substantial investment in scarce agency resources
- The resistance of service providers to evaluation, since they already have confidence that the care they are providing is high quality and is having a positive impact on clients
- The fact that evaluation reports have most often not been written for practitioners, nor have they usually been directly relevant or applicable to daily practice concerns.

These reasons, along with numerous others that undoubtedly could be added to this list, provide persuasive justifications many agencies use to ignore monitoring and evaluation activities. In fact, these reasons are so convincing and pervasive that it is rare for ongoing programs to undertake evaluative efforts. Most agencies are struggling to provide the needed services to their clientele while remaining within a specific budget. The thought of placing additional resources into program evaluation is not only unappealing, but in many cases objectionable. Using scarce resources on efforts that have not demonstrated high payoff to the organization has not been considered good management by many program administrators and staff.

There are, however, several important reasons for conducting evaluative studies in case management programs, including:

- The need to comply with agency regulators (although not the best reason, it may realistically provide the highest motivation)
- The need to demonstrate agency accomplishments and effectiveness to funding sources
- The need to improve the practice of agency personnel including: methods of allocating services, more accurate targeting of clients, and enhanced supervision of case managers.

Improving agency practice is the most compelling reason to conduct monitoring and evaluative activities. Practitioners may often assume that their current practice is the most beneficial to clients. In some cases, however, other methods may prove to be superior. The objective of this section is to provide case management agencies with methods to monitor and evaluate the effectiveness of their programs. If evaluation activities are not designed to provide useful information to agency personnel, there is little incentive for agencies, particularly given existing resource constraints, to initiate such activities.

In the following chapters, questions that emphasize issues of practice effectiveness are raised. In many areas, the evaluative activities described can be completed by agency staff. In other areas, consultation from outside experts may be needed. At the outset, however, the agency must recognize the importance of maintaining active responsibility for the overall evaluation effort. Integrating monitoring and evaluation activities into ongoing agency operations means that the organization must link its planning, evaluation, and quality assurance components. Furthermore, adequate information and information systems will be the key ingredients for successful evaluative activities.

APPROACHES TO EVALUATION AND QUALITY ASSURANCE

It is important to differentiate between three distinct concepts: quality, evaluation, and quality assurance. The premise of this book is that a major objective of case management agencies is the provision of quality services to the most needy individuals in the most efficient and effective manner possible. Evidence of good quality care is provided through the combined functions of evaluation and quality assurance (Applebaum, 1989).

Evaluation poses the basic question of whether the services that are delivered have had their intended effects. Do the individuals that receive a particular service(s) do better than those not receiving such care? Toothpaste commercials on television are an example of this approach. For example, do individuals who brush with a particular toothpaste do better (as measured by the number of cavities) than individuals not brushing with that toothpaste? Do individuals receiving case-managed care do better than those who do not?

Once it has been established that a particular service or product does, indeed, result in the expected outcomes, it becomes possible to address quality assurance. Quality assurance asks the question: How can this beneficial outcome be assured across time and across a variety of settings and case managers? Quality assurance involves two major components. First, the product or service must be operationally defined, and second, precise standards must be developed. For example, in case management, it is necessary to develop practice standards in order to know exactly what good case management looks like (not an easy task). Until the service or product is defined and the standards are established, it is not possible to ensure quality. After practice standards have been developed, the quality assurance process is used to monitor whether the service as delivered complies with the standards. Thus, quality assurance means "compliance to standards" (Crosby, 1979).

Combining evaluation (knowing the outcomes of a service) and quality assurance (knowing that the service is implemented in a consistent manner as designed) results in a comprehensive approach to ensuring high quality care. Detailed discussion of quality assurance and evaluation are presented in Chapters 6 and 7, respectively.

It is important to emphasize that the selection of specific evaluative and quality assurance techniques must be tailored to the individual circumstances of the agency involved. Factors such as size of the program, resources available, program objectives, funding source requirements, and perceived effectiveness all help to determine appropriate monitoring and evaluative techniques. Needless to say, no one best approach exists or should be prescribed for all case management programs.

Experience suggests that there is confusion surrounding the concepts of program evaluation and quality assurance. Often, evaluation and quality assurance definitions and components are used interchangeably. In the following section, a detailed description of the way in which program evaluation and quality assurance functions have been operationalized will be discussed.

Operationalizing Evaluation

Efforts to conduct program evaluation can be classified into three categories:

- *descriptive measures* and indicators that can provide a description of program components
- *program review* that provides a qualitative review of case management practice
- *program impact studies* that assess the extent to which specific outcomes have been accomplished for clients receiving case management service.

Each of these is discussed and summarized in Table 5–1.

TABLE 5-1 Evaluation Approaches for Examining Case Management Effectiveness

Approach description	Strengths	Limitations
Descriptive measures Measures and indicators that provide a description of program components. Serve dual purpose as quality assurance performance indicators and as description of program for more extensive evaluation.	Generally straightforward to collect and measure.	These measures do require some type of information system. Do not provide conclusive evaluative information about program outcomes, only indicators.
Program review Provides a qualitative review of case management practice, emphasizing a review of processes performed by case managers.	Allows organization to review actual practice of case managers, and to make judgments about quality of case management activities.	Does not provide conclusive evaluation information about the effectiveness of program outcomes.
Program impact Examines specific outcomes for those receiving case-managed care. Relies on experimental design where program clients are compared to a nonprogram group.	The most powerful way to examine program impacts. Provides program with information about specific outcomes.	Generally the most difficult type of evaluation approach to implement. Requires more expertise, resources, and involves more burden to clients.

Descriptive Measures or Indicators. The creation of descriptive measures or indicators is an essential first step in evaluating any program. Their purpose is to clarify key elements of the program so that the nature of the services provided by the agency are clearly understood. Documentation of the program components can be accomplished through both quantitative indicators and qualitative indicators. An example of a quantitative program indicator would be the length of time that it took to complete an assessment after a new client was referred to the program. If, for example, the elapsed time from the point of referral to the completion of an assessment was three months, agency staff might conclude that they were not operating at an acceptable level, given the needs of the client population the program is designed to serve. Very often, however, agencies do not know how long it takes to accomplish many programmatic functions. A more qualitative approach might involve interviews with key referral sources to check on the adequacy of the referral process.

There are numerous indicators that agencies can use to describe and document program activities. These indicators do not address program outcomes; however, they can provide essential information about program operations. Descriptive measures serve two primary purposes for a program. First, they serve as indicators of good practice in their own right, and second, they provide the necessary foundation for other evaluative approaches. In the next chapter, a series of indicators is presented and analyzed in terms of how they could be used.

Descriptive indicators have the advantage of being conceptually straightforward and, by and large, easy to define. Information items that can serve as descriptive indicators have already been collected or are continuously collected in many organizations. For example, many organizations currently collect information on the type of referral sources and the characteristics of clients. These indicators would not require that the agency employ individuals with substantial evaluation experience, since the indicators rely on routine program information that is generated by personnel.

The major disadvantage of the descriptive indicators approach is that the agency must have an information system, either manual or automated, to receive, tabulate, and review information in a systematic fashion. If an information system does not exist, it must be developed. In most cases, this means that an agency must reevaluate the information it currently collects and processes. Given the inherent conflict between the amount of paperwork that agency staff can manage and the amount of information requested by planners and evaluators, consideration of what constitutes necessary information requirements is an important issue. Experience demonstrates that requiring program staff to spend considerable time completing paperwork without providing them with the benefits of that information is almost always a recipe for failure. Integrating information requirements for evaluation and planning, as well as ensuring participation of personnel from all levels in these critical activities are two crucial elements of successful evaluation, quality assurance, and planning. Unfortunately, a considerable amount of staff time and resources are required to thoroughly develop these functions. Especially in times of scarce resources, this means that funds for planning, evaluative, and quality assurance activities will compete for support with direct service activities. This is support that might be taken away from direct client service or case management support tasks.

Program Review Approach. The program review approach involves systematic review to assure quality of case management activities. Here a "best practice" strategy is used in which case manager activities are compared to professional program standards. For example, in some agencies a program audit is used in which a sample of cases is selected for review by a panel of independent professionals. The panel of experts, for example, might then be asked to review the care plans for sample cases and compare these plans to the client assessment data. Problems that were documented in the initial assessment but not addressed in the care plan would be identified in this review. This information could then become part of the agency's supervisory process. For example, if certain case managers systematically omitted working with informal caregivers, or failed to address mental health problems, this program review could be used to identify these patterns and would be valuable for improving comprehensiveness of client care plans.

Another type of program review activity involves independent experts who accompany assessors on initial client interviews. By recording their observations on a duplicate form, experts can provide feedback to case managers about how they conducted the assessment process. This strategy can be of particular value when the program is attempting to ensure that case managers from different disciplines identify the same client problems. For instance, this approach could be used to assure that the case managers with social work training identify client problems that might require medical attention, and conversely that nurse case managers address nonmedical problems such as psychosocial functioning. Program review is particularly valuable as a training technique. Systematic review provides information about whether comparable, uniform assessments are conducted by case managers. This approach clearly relies on the development of practice standards for case management.

Program review data do not provide definitive evaluative information about program impact. The program review approach does, however, provide important information about the quality of the case management and can function as an important quality assurance and supervisory technique. The major advantage of the program review strategy is that it can be developed for relatively modest costs. Although the approach does require some expertise such as determining the appropriate number of cases to review and how cases should be selected, in general it can be designed and administered by agency personnel. Program review activities that utilize external experts also have the advantage of injecting new insights into ongoing program operations.

There are, however, important limitations to the program review approach. First and foremost is that this method does not always adequately capture the intricacies of long-term care case management. A "paper review" comparison of assessment data and care plans may not accurately reflect the complexities of a particular case. For example, excluding a particular problem from the care plan may have been the best practice decision based on the dynamics of a client's situation. For example, although a client may be experiencing mental health problems, this need could possibly be excluded from the plan until a later time because of resistance from the client and family. In addition, as a result of the complexities of case management practice, it may prove difficult for professional reviewers to agree on one "best practice" approach to providing care. Cost can also be a factor in this approach. Staff time in selecting cases for review and the cost of professional reviewer time should not be underestimated. If professional reviewers require reimbursement (volunteers can be recruited in some cases), agency funds will also be required. Thus, although the program review method provides a mechanism for evaluating programs, it is not without limitations.

Program Impact Evaluation. The program impact approach is designed to answer the question of whether the case management program, as provided, affects clients differently than an alternative model of care. In this type of evaluation, a specific group of individuals receiving the case management services is compared to a nonprogram group with similar characteristics and experiences. The program impact approach requires a control group not receiving the program services in order to compare this group to those receiving program services.

The program impact strategy has been used in most of the community care demonstration projects reviewed earlier. For example, in the National Channeling Demonstration, individuals who were eligible for the project were randomly assigned either to receive services from the Channeling program or to receive services that were normally available in the community. Throughout an 18-month time period, researchers monitored outcomes for all clients in the Channeling study. Comparisons on outcomes such as mortality, nursing home and hospital use, and client life quality were examined for both groups. The outcomes of the channeling program were evaluated by comparing results for both groups on specific outcome measures, such as rate of nursing home use.

The program impact approach provides a mechanism for examining specific client outcomes. A study using proper evaluation design procedures can address a question of fundamental and ultimate importance: Do individuals receiving program services function better, worse, or the same as similar individuals not receiving the services? Although the other program evaluation approaches discussed previously can provide insight regarding the program as implemented, they cannot directly address client outcomes.

Despite the advantages of program impact evaluation, this approach also has some major limitations. Designing and implementing an experimental study requires substantial effort on the part of the agency staff. In most cases, outside expertise will be necessary to design, implement, and analyze the study, thus requiring substantial resources. In addition to agency costs, program impact evaluation may prove to be more burdensome to applicants and clients. If well implemented, an evaluation of this nature will be a major effort for an agency. Thus, although impact evaluation is the most rigorous evaluative approach, several barriers make it difficult to implement.

Quality Assurance

Although quality assurance has been discussed considerably in the acute and long-term care institutional health arenas, it has received little attention in case management and community-based services. Recently, community based care providers have recognized the importance of quality assurance activities, and the emphasis on quality assurance has increased appreciably.

Approaches to ensuring the quality of care have traditionally been classified into three categories: structure, process, and outcome (Donabedian, 1966). A summary of these approaches is presented in Table 5–2.

Structural Strategy. Structural strategies for quality assurance analyze the organizational framework for service delivery to ensure that services are of high quality. Structural methods assume that individuals or agencies meeting certain structural standards can provide the expected level of quality care. The structural approach, which includes elements such as agency certification, individual licensure, training standards, bonding of employees, staffing ratios, and professional credentialing, essentially measures the capacity of the organization to provide care. It is based on the assumption that if providers

TABLE 5–2 Quality Assurance Approaches

Approach description	Strengths	Limitations
Structural strategy Structural efforts to ensure quality have generally examined the agencies' *capacity* to provide care—are they licensed, do employees meet training standards, etc.	Such efforts are by and large straightforward to measure and routinely available	These measures are indicators of capacity, but do not necessarily ensure quality
Process strategy Observes service provision in order to assess whether service is provided at an acceptable level of practice	Allows direct practice to be reviewed in a systematic manner to ensure that common practice standards are being followed	Requires professional agreement on determining good practice; greater subjectivity can exist in process review
Outcomes strategy Attempts to focus on what happens to clients after the service has been provided. Does the desired outcome occur?		Monitoring service effects on client outcomes must be a key quality assurance component Measurement of outcomes can be difficult. Adequate application of technology can be a problem.

meet the established requirements of their field that it is likely that good quality care will be provided.

Structural measures have been the dominant mode used to ensure quality of care. A major reason for this heavy reliance on structural methods is that, by and large, they are easy to measure and data are routinely collected in these areas. For example, it may be difficult to know how well a case manager or service provider is doing on the job, but it is relatively easy to ascertain whether they are trained or licensed.

Although the structural approach has been used widely in efforts to ensure quality, it is recognized that quality assurance strategies can not rely solely on these measures. Structural indicators are viewed as necessary first steps, but are not sufficient, in and of themselves, to ensure that a service will be of high quality.

Process Strategy. The process approach examines the way in which a particular service is provided compared to acceptable levels of practice. This strategy assumes that, with the establishment of specific standards, a trained individual can observe the service being provided and judge whether that service is being provided properly. For example, if one monitors the care provided by a home health aide, a professional can judge if the home health aide task, such as transferring the client from a bed to a wheelchair, is performed properly.

The process approach requires identifying or developing practice standards of care. Process review can be accomplished through record reviews, personal observations, personal interviews, or a combination of these methods. It provides a direct review of practice and, as such, can provide specific and useful feedback about the care provided. The limitation of this approach is that it relies on professional wisdom, which is not always sufficient. For example, bloodletting could have been performed according to the standard of the day, but it still would not have been an effective practice. Similar types of practice uncertainties undoubtedly exist today.

Outcome Strategy. Outcome strategy focuses on what happens to the client after the service has been provided. Does the person receiving the care maintain or improve in the area of care provided? For example, does the patient under the care of a physician improve in the condition being treated? Is the nursing home resident well nourished, clean, socially active, and satisfied with the care received? Are the case-managed clients receiving the correct package of services such that their major care needs are met? Under outcome strategies, the expected and desirable outcomes of service delivery must be identified so that the care received can be reviewed according to these standards.

The outcome approach has as its major strength the provision of direct information about the client's condition. As such, it is far superior to the structure and process techniques, which serve as precursors to quality. However, outcome assessment has two limitations. First, the actual outcome for a particular service can often be difficult to define, measure, and collect. Client judgment of service quality can be particularly difficult to operationalize. Collecting and recording this type of information requires considerable effort as well. The second limitation has to do with the methodology traditionally used under the outcome approach. Outcome efforts have generally focused on the care of individual clients or groups of clients without the benefit of experimental design methods normally used in impact evaluation. As a result, it can be difficult for the outcome approach to distinguish between the negative effects that result from poor quality service and expected deterioration of the client being served. This is a particular problem when serving a population of people with long-term care needs.

QUALITY ASSURANCE EFFORTS

Several recent efforts implemented in the long-term care arena have attempted to integrate structural, process, and outcome approaches. In a recently completed quality assurance demonstration project in Ohio (Applebaum, Atchley, McGinnis, Bare, 1988), client outcomes in such areas as living environment, satisfaction with care, adequacy of personal care, and hygiene and nutritional status were examined as part of the quality assurance process. In this project, random home visits were conducted each month on a sample of clients. If, based on a visit, the clients' condition was found to be substandard (poor physical condition, personal care not performed, homemaking tasks not completed), an examination of the care being provided was then performed. Quality assurance activities examined these outcomes in the context of the structure and processes of care provision. In this manner, outcomes served as indicators in a balanced quality assurance system.

The newly revised nursing home survey procedures, which attempt to focus on client outcomes, provide another example of this effort. Under this approach, nursing home surveyors examine client outcomes for a series of health and social factors (decubitus ulcers, falls, bruises, satisfaction with care) in an effort to assess the quality of care. In cases where the client's condition is below standard, a careful review of structural and process indicators of the resident's care is completed in an effort to link these aspects of care delivery with resident outcomes.

Under the previous nursing home survey approach, surveyors focused on a series of structural and process-related roles, with little focus on client outcomes. Structural roles, such as use of marked fire exits, kitchen cleanliness, and locked cabinets dominated the review process. Although these dimensions were not unimportant, they were far from sufficient to ensure quality of care. Thus, the revised survey process has attempted to create more of a balanced emphasis on structure, process, and outcomes. Whether this objective is reached in the new survey process has yet to be determined.

Incorporating outcomes into the quality assurance process has not been a common practice in case-managed community-based care. However, integrating structural, process, and outcome efforts is essential for the development of a good quality assurance system. Structural components, such as in-home worker training and supervision, are useful system concerns, but these types of measures alone are not sufficient to ensure quality.

BLENDING QUALITY ASSURANCE AND PROGRAM EVALUATION

The previous discussion of quality assurance and program evaluation approaches highlights the fact that both differences and similarities exist between these activities. Quality assurance has focused considerably on structural measures to ensure that services will be of good quality, while program evaluation has not generally emphasized this area. Process review has been used in both evaluation and quality assurance, although it has been a more common technique of quality assurance. Outcome approaches have also been used in both areas, but with one major difference. The outcomes strategy in quality assurance has until recently been quite limited and focused on the individual client or client group without the benefit of experimental design. The use of outcomes in program evaluation in conjunction with an experimental design has been more common, although even in this area such an approach has been used most often in demonstrations or pilot projects rather than in ongoing programs.

Comparing these two areas suggests that, in many instances, elements of quality assurance and program evaluation are interchangeable. For instance, a descriptive evaluation component, such as the length of time taken to provide services, could also be defined as an element of a quality assurance system. As noted, process review techniques under program evaluation and quality assurance also overlap. Although there are some differences between program evaluation and quality assurance concepts and terminology, it is our contention that the key elements of both must be combined as part of an agency's strategy for providing quality services. The combination of these approaches requires developing the type of overall agency planning and evaluation strategy that is discussed in the following section.

Principles for Conducting Agency-Based Program Evaluation and Quality Assurance

It should be emphasized that the overall responsibility for program planning, monitoring, and evaluation activities should rest within the agency. Although using outside consultants may be appropriate and perhaps essential in certain circumstances, the agency must retain ultimate responsibility for its own activities. To this end, the following practice principles are recommended:

- To design a useful evaluation and monitoring system, an organization should link its planning, administrative, and evaluation practices together.

- An individual or individuals within the agency should have the primary responsibility for the planning and evaluation process. Outside consultants may be essential in the design and examination of planning and evaluative processes, but evaluation activities should not be treated as external problems to be handled by the consultants.

- In order to design a strong model of planning and evaluation, an organization should involve a broad range of participants from within the agency.

- Agency administrative staff must have a strong commitment to designing an integrated planning and evaluation process. Adequate resources must be allocated to planning and evaluation if these efforts are to be successful.

Taken together, these principles form an alternative model for planning, monitoring, and evaluating agency programs. In order to be meaningful to the agency, an ongoing quality assurance and program evaluation system should be guided by the model presented below. Each of the model's principles is discussed.

Link Planning, Administrative, and Evaluation Practices Together. This first recommendation focuses on how evaluation and monitoring activities fit into the overall planning and administrative activities of the organization. Evaluative efforts cannot be a separate activity within the agency, but must be an integral part of program administration. In order for monitoring and evaluation activities to be meaningful to an organization, the agency must carefully examine planning and administrative needs. Collecting data, using information systems, and implementing specific evaluation activities, must be designed and implemented in the context of overall agency needs. This is not to suggest that single evaluative components cannot have positive effects on case management practice, but to highlight the importance of an integrated approach. For example, developing a recording process to examine the length of time it took the agency to provide services to the client (elapsed time) could provide important information. A client recording system, however, should fit into the larger data needs of the agency as part of a comprehensive planning and administrative model. A major concern frequently expressed by case managers is the amount of paperwork they are asked to complete. In these circumstances, it is important that the agency carefully examine data collection forms and elements across the organization before adding to the paperwork burden already carried by many case managers. In order to integrate evaluation and monitoring activities, agency staff have to understand how administrative components and procedures, as well as planning processes, can be designed to incorporate program evaluation tasks.

In discussing the integration of monitoring and evaluation activities, it is essential to highlight the importance of developing an adequate system for processing information. Many local agencies have not developed a strong mechanism for recording, manipulating, or presenting evaluative information. It is even more unusual for an organization to coordinate planning, quality assurance, and program evaluation needs in an effort to create a comprehensive information system. In fact, there are numerous horror stories of unsuccessful attempts to develop computerized information systems. Searching for the right information system is not the focus of this section; however, recognizing the importance of processing information in a useful way is critical to any agency interested in quality assurance and evaluation techniques.

Assign Primary Responsibility Within the Agency. Responsibility is one of the key elements of this model. *Agency staff* have to *maintain* overall *responsibility* for the planning and evaluative process. A common problem with both evaluative and planning activities is that agency staff often do not see these two efforts as integral parts of agency practice. Because managers and practitioners often focus primarily on day-to-day program operations and frequently have to worry about the daily brush fire, it is difficult to allocate sufficient time to planning and evaluative needs. Frequently, however, planning and evaluative needs *become* brush fires. This can occur, for example, when a major funding source asks for a quality assurance plan or an evaluation of a specific program. Where agencies have become involved in evaluation and monitoring activities, it is not uncommon for either outside consultants or nonprogram staff to be primary actors in the evaluation process. In the absence of substantial participation from program staff, this approach often causes problems, both in terms of data collection and in terms of relevance of results. In order to avoid these problems, it is strongly recommended that overall responsibility (or at least strong involvement) remain with program and administrative personnel who are directly accountable for program activities.

In designing and planning quality assurance and evaluative activities, it is often necessary to use outside consultants. Since most of the agency personnel are involved either directly or indirectly with providing services to clients, it is not surprising that many organizations and their staff have limited experience with evaluation design, information systems, and models of planning.

When consultants are involved, several important points about their selection and use should be kept in mind. First, there are many different ways to obtain consultation for evaluative or quality assurance purposes. In some locations, there are universities that may have useful resources. Graduate students and faculty can be used as outside experts. In most universities, faculty are expected to provide community service. Involvement in various agencies' evaluation and quality assurance activities can be a vehicle for faculty to fulfill their responsibility to provide community service. Faculty are also interested in writing research articles. Providing faculty with access to program data is an attraction that agency staff should not underestimate. A second set of resources may be available in many communities through the local United Way or United Appeal umbrella organization. Throughout the country, these agencies have emphasized integrative planning and often have consultation services available for local agencies. Finally, there are a number of private consulting organizations and individuals that may have useful expertise.

When an organization is exploring the use of outside consultants, several important points should be emphasized. While there may be a number of knowledgeable and excellent consultants available, there are also individuals and organizations with very limited expertise. In choosing a consultant, be sure to find out the type of work that the company and individuals have done in the past. Ask for examples of previous work including proposals, reports, and executive summaries. Contact other agencies with whom the consultant has worked. Get a specific bid on what needs to be done, rather than an open-ended consulting agreement that reimburses the contractor for whatever time is spent. Selecting the best consultant is a very important decision. A bad decision here will most likely create significant problems far into the future.

Once a competent consultant has been identified, it is dangerous to assume that everything is automatically under control. Most experienced consultants try to help agency staff structure their time so as to maximize their use. This, however, is something that takes a substantial amount of effort. Many of the issues that are faced in laying out a planning, evaluation, and monitoring model involve considerable discussion with and among organizational staff. If agencies have not assigned internal staff to assume primary responsibility, many of the tasks that should be performed by internal personnel will be left needlessly to the consultant. These circumstances should be avoided for two reasons: process (many important discussions will be lost) and cost. In some instances, it will be important to have an outside expert available to help facilitate meetings. However, this kind of involvement should be carefully calculated. The proper consulting role must be negotiated and agreed upon by internal staff with primary responsibility for these activities, agency management, and the consultant. Setting priorities governing how, when, and where consultation will be used is an essential task. Using outside consultation can save time, money, and improve the product significantly; however, this outcome requires considerable effort.

Involve a Broad Range of Quality Assurance Staff. A key element of an integrated planning and evaluation model is a mechanism for including staff from units and departments across the organization. An evaluation strategy developed collaboratively by case managers, supervisors, case aides, data entry personnel, administrative staff, and other agency personnel is critical to the process. The chances that an evaluation approach is going to be adopted will be increased if the process is developed, at least in part, by agency staff. These are the key individuals who are ultimately going to be involved in collecting and utilizing evaluation information. There are countless examples of programs collecting data that are useful neither for agency practice nor for evaluation purposes. In this circumstance, the process will prove to be time consuming, nonproductive, and will eventually atrophy from lack of use.

Using a committee that includes representatives from each component of the agency is one mechanism that can help ensure broad based involvement. This type of involvement means that it will take longer to develop an agency evaluation strategy. If, however, the process increases staff commitment to evaluation activities, it will be of considerable value in the long run.

Administrative Staff Must Have a Strong Commitment to an Integrated Planning and Evaluation Process. As the previous recommendations imply, implementing a comprehensive model of planning, monitoring, and evaluation requires a considerable amount of human and financial resources. Examining the planning, administrative, and evaluation needs of an organization is a major undertaking. Including a broad range of agency staff requires an even greater investment of time and resources. Furthermore, using outside consultants can also require a large investment on the part of the agency. This includes both economic costs and staff time, since staff time is needed in order to use consultants properly. The key point is that developing and implementing a comprehensive planning, evaluation, and monitoring strategy requires a major initial investment and an ongoing maintenance effort. Agency staff must carefully assess their needs and resources in determining a strategy. Even if a more limited approach is undertaken, considerable organizational investment will be necessary to think strategically about where the agency wants to be in the future in the area of planning, monitoring, and evaluation.

A final principle involves the administrative commitment to the planning and evaluation process. If those individuals responsible for organizational management are not committed to the planning and evaluation process, in all probability little serious activity will be undertaken in this area. As noted, a process of this nature requires the commitment of agency staff and financial resources. Without allocating a sufficient amount of each, it will be extremely difficult for an agency to conduct effective planning and evaluative activities. Although planning and evaluation activities must be discussed throughout the agency, managers who set the organizational tone and provide leadership will largely determine the degree to which the agency emphasizes these critical activities.

Chapter 6

Quality Assurance of Case-Managed Care

The following two chapters examine a series of key questions that are central to evaluating and ensuring the quality of case management practice. This chapter focuses on quality assurance and descriptive evaluation issues, and the next chapter explores program evaluation *outcome* questions. While both of these activities are critical monitoring programs, there is a clear and important distinction between them. Quality assurance or descriptive evaluation approaches provide an indicator of quality and effectiveness without the benefit of a comparison group. The comparative approach uses the experiences of at least one additional group (a control or comparison group) to evaluate program effectiveness.

In the quality assurance approach, the focus on client outcomes is from an individual case perspective. For example, if a review of client conditions identifies an individual(s) with declining physical functioning or an abnormal number of hospital admissions, or low satisfaction with care, these outcomes trigger an examination of the care received. Using this approach, the outcomes serve as indicators of the process of delivering care. In some instances, the care might have been provided properly even though the outcome was negative. In other instances, a negative client outcome could clearly be a result of poor quality care. The key point here is that in a quality assurance approach, the unit of analysis is the individual case.

Descriptive evaluation examines data in an aggregate manner as well. Under this approach, similar outcomes may be examined; however, the unit of analysis is primarily the group rather than individual clients. Analysis of group data is then used as an indicator of aggregate program performance. For example, if 75 percent of the respondents on a client satisfaction survey reported that they were not satisfied with the care received, this result would provide important evaluative information about the program. As in the client-focused approach, the agency would want to link outcomes with other descriptive and process monitoring techniques.

The *comparative* outcome approach is distinctly different from the *descriptive* evaluation or quality assurance strategies. The comparative outcome approach asks the question: What would happen to program participants in the absence of this particular program? Effects on specific individuals are not the focus of this technique. Rather, the effects on the entire group as compared to a group of nonprogram clients is the unit of study. This strategy, based on experimental design, is commonly called impact evaluation is explored in Chapter 7.

A series of questions about the practice of case management provide the framework for our examination of quality assurance (See Table 6–1).

These questions focus solely on whether case management activities are implemented according to design. As such, they are part of a

TABLE 6–1 Descriptive Evaluation and Quality Assurance Questions

Question	Data source
(1) How well does the agency implement program eligibility and targeting criteria?	compare initial assessment with criteria use of reinterview to validate data collection
(2) Are assessment and care planning functions completed in a timely fashion in accordance with practice standards?	audit review strategy track client progress through record system formalized qualitative review
(3) To what extent do the service plans meet client needs?	client record system professional program review financial control system
(4) Are the service plans actually implemented?	systematic use of monitoring strategies—provider reports, case manager checks use of different data sources to reassess and record client's condition

set of quality assurance activities designed to assess whether the intervention is in compliance with particular program standards. Quality assurance questions do not address topics concerning the direct effects of case-managed care on clients. (These are discussed in the subsequent chapter on outcomes.)

- How well does the agency implement program eligibility and targeting criteria?
- Does the agency complete structured client assessment and formalized care plans in a timely fashion?
- To what extent do service plans meet client needs?
- Are the service plans designed actually implemented?
- Are clients satisfied with the case-managed care received?

[A standard is defined as a clear statement of an acceptable level of care that results in a desired quality end. *Criteria* are measurable indicators that operationalize the intent of the standard (Adapted from Manual of Nursing Quality Assurance, Rowland & Rowland, p. 2.8, 1987).]

As noted, quality assurance asks the question: Is the service being provided as designed? In order to have a quality assurance system it is thus essential for a case management agency to have an established set of standards for each of the services to be monitored. If service definitions do not exist, it is not possible in our view for quality assurance activities to be implemented. The development of standards in case-managed community-based care programs has presented a formidable challenge. It has been far easier to "identify quality when you see it," than it has been to establish clearly defined standards of care. For example, although a set of care standards could be developed for the provision of personal care (i.e., proper techniques for lifting and transferring a person), certain components of the personal care tasks are more difficult to define. A smile or touch or a kind word may make a difference to the client, but these important aspects of quality are not easily defined or measured as part of service standards. Even so, continued development and refinement of service standards and criteria are essential elements of a quality assurance system.

The monitoring questions that are examined in this chapter are examples of questions that provide evidence concerning whether the service is being provided according to the design. Because differences in program standards may vary across providers (depending upon such factors as type of client served, services available, caseload size, and geographical differences), individual programs will need to tailor standards and monitoring questions to specific programs. The questions addressed in this section are illustrative of the type of questions that could be identified by case management providers.

HOW WELL DOES THE AGENCY IMPLEMENT PROGRAM ENTRANCE CRITERIA?

One key question case management programs face is simply how clients enter the program. Given the limited number of clients who can actually be served, agencies must make important decisions about how to equitably allocate scarce service resources. Although most case management programs screen clients at entry, a final eligibility determination is performed by the case manager. Here, case managers serve in a dual role, as client advocates and as system gatekeepers. Thus, the evaluative question is: How well do case managers implement the program eligibility criteria? (Or, from a quality assurance perspective, are the established criteria for program eligibility being followed according to the design?)

One approach that can be used to examine how well eligibility criteria are applied is to compare client characteristics at the baseline (the initial) assessment (the point at which eligibility is determined) with the program entry criteria. In order to make this comparison, a case management program would need to list program entry requirements comprehensively and then make sure that the same data items are included in the assessment process. For example, in the Channeling Demonstration, individuals were required to:

- demonstrate a functional disability as measured by their performance in activities of daily living
- have unmet need for services
- be over age 65
- in some sites, be eligible for Medicare

These criteria were then examined for every client entering the program at each of the 10 Channeling sites. Findings indicated that in approximately 86 percent of the cases, clients were reported to have met the program entry criteria. Although program entry and baseline assessment comparisons in this example were made for each of the 10 channeling sites, the analysis could be performed in a number of ways—for individual case managers within a single organization, for satellite offices within a large city, or for regions throughout a state.

Although comparisons of this nature are generally straightforward, one potential methodological concern involves the accuracy of the baseline eligibility data. Since eligibility determination is based on assessments completed by case managers, there is some concern that the recorded forms may not accurately reflect client status, and that case managers, in their advocacy role, record the characteristics clients need to become eligible for the program. If this occurs, a problem with validity of the eligibility data is present. There are, however, research methods that can test whether this problem exists. For example, in order to examine the validity of the eligibility determination process, a reinterview assessment using independent reviewers can be conducted for a sample of cases. The Channeling experience with this approach indicated that, although there were statistically significant differences between initial assessments and reinterviews on a number of items,[1] these differences changed program eligibility decisions in only a small number of cases (less than 10 percent). Furthermore, these findings indicated that changes in eligibility decisions after reinterview were not consistent in one direction or another. For example, the applicant was not always found ineligible at the reinterview. As a result of this analysis, there was some confidence that the original data recorded by case managers was, in fact, valid.

Those programs with managed-care responsibilities, such as the S/HMO projects, must also monitor client characteristics upon entry. In fact, because the S/HMO requires a balanced risk pool, it is necessary to ensure a mixture of frail and well enrollees. Thus, a system to monitor characteristics of applicants had to be established in each of the four project sites. This type of validation analysis is especially critical when the case management provider is at financial risk. Validation analysis not only substantiates that the entry criteria are being observed, but also ensures objectivity in assessment data, supports good clinical practice, and assures that the balance in the risk pool is maintained. There are, however, some disadvantages to a reinterview approach. Most importantly, more burden is placed on the clients, since they are asked to complete two assessments in a relatively short time period. Other problems with the approach involve its accuracy given the passage of time and the frequent instability of client conditions. Many clients with chronic impairments enter community care programs during a period of crisis. Their conditions may change rapidly. In some cases, even the location of the assessment and reassessment interview changes, most often from hospital to home. The key point is that close attention must be given to the validity of the

---

[1]Statistically significant means that in this case there is a 95 percent chance that differences of this size are due to actual differences in the interviews rather than chance.

reassessment information being collected. Several factors can affect the validity of these data.

Analysis of this baseline assessment and program entry criteria comparison must take into account that the interpretation of findings is program specific. For example, one program may consider an 86 percent eligibility an indicator of strict enforcement, while another may see this as unacceptable implementation of program criteria. Although interpretations of outcomes are subject to political and contextual factors, the comparative process does provide important program information. If, for example, only 25 percent of the clientele were meeting the eligibility criteria, agency staff should consider changing entrance procedures. The main point is that without clearly stated, *objective* eligibility criteria, program administrators will not be able to compare entrance requirements with actual client characteristics. Without the capacity to make this comparison, case management programs will not be able to assess the validity of their process for allocating services.

Since the population in need of community-based long-term care will only increase in the future, the validity of program entry data will require closer attention in case management programs. Community agencies are receiving more and more requests for services from an increasingly disabled population, often making it difficult to decide which clients to serve. In some cases, homemaker agencies are being forced to withdraw services from their less disabled clientele. Recent policy developments such as the prospective payment hospital reimbursement system (DRGs) and cutbacks in home health benefits, combined with continued demographic changes, mean that service allocation decisions are becoming more and more critical.

A final point must be emphasized. While comparison of client entry characteristics to program eligibility criteria may be a useful process evaluative strategy, it does not address the question of whether the criteria being used are correct. Even if clients meet program entry criteria in every case, it is not accurate to conclude that the program is, in fact, serving the most appropriate target population. This issue will be addressed in greater detail in a subsequent section.

ARE STRUCTURED ASSESSMENTS AND FORMALIZED CARE PLANS COMPLETED IN A TIMELY FASHION?

State-of-the-art case management practice includes several key practice components discussed earlier in this volume. Determining whether these critical activities have been completed in a timely fashion is an important indicator of program efficiency. In a number of programs, case management standards actually include practice norms or standards for the completion of these activities. Although one would hope that human service organizations would respond quickly to the needs of applicants, many agencies do not record this information and, therefore, do not know how long it takes them to respond to client need. Several quality assurance approaches have been developed to examine the timeliness-of-response issue. Three of these strategies are:

- an audit review strategy
- a client record reporting strategy
- a formalized qualitative review.

Audit Review Strategy

The audit review strategy involves a review of client files by independent or supervisory personnel. The audit generally reviews program assessment and care planning instruments for timeliness and completeness. For example, in the National Channeling study, project personnel established a program standard that clients should receive an initial assessment within seven working days after referral. The audit review focused on both completion and timeliness of assessments. One of the Channeling sites found that 70 percent of the assessments were fully completed within the specified time period. The audit review strategy does not provide information regarding accuracy of client assessments, but it does provide important program performance information to the agency.

A key issue in the audit review approach is whether the audit should be conducted on the entire caseload or whether a sample is adequate. If a sample is adequate, how large a sample is necessary? To answer this question, agency staff might require some technical advice, since there is no clear-cut rule for making this decision. There are, however, several important principles that can guide this process.

To address the question of whether a sample of cases or the entire caseload should be used, program personnel will first need to examine the number of clients served over a specified time period (1 year, for example). If the program is small (50 clients per year) then a sample may not be necessary. If, on the other hand, a program is serving several thousand individuals, a sample will be necessary to make audit review feasible.

Several important points should be emphasized regarding determination of sample size. The object of taking a sample is to get as accurate a picture of the entire caseload as possible without the expense of reviewing every record or interviewing every client. The lack of accurate representation in a sample is referred to as sampling error. Research textbooks are filled with classic cases in which sampling errors have caused pollsters to misinterpret public opinion, such as the famous prediction of Dewey over Truman in the 1948 Presidential election. In evaluation research, failure to sample correctly can lead to misleading or incorrect conclusions about the program under study.

In considering sample size for an audit review, two major factors must be considered. First, the number of cases sampled should be large enough so that meaningful comparisons can be made. The second and most important factor when considering sample size involves selecting at least the minimum sample size needed to represent accurately the population from which the sample is drawn. Evaluators perform detailed sample size calculations based on a series of statistical concepts and assumptions including the confidence level required and the variation of the responses (known as the standard error). A thorough understanding of these concepts is required for accurate sample size calculations. If necessary, case management programs can use consultants to help arrive at an optimum sample size. Although "rules of thumb" leave room for error, one convention on sample size discussed in the literature (Grinnell, 1981) recommends a sample of one-tenth (1/10) the size of the total client population being sampled. In agencies with a total caseload size below 150, it is recommended that the percentage be increased to ensure that no fewer than 15 clients are reviewed.

Sampling errors can occur for two separate but often related reasons: first, errors in the process of selecting the sample, and second, because the sample size is too small. For the evaluation and monitoring activities discussed in this book, the sampling process *must* use some type of *random* sample. This means that cases are selected *only by chance*. Selecting cases through any other mechanism, such as allowing supervisors to choose or having case managers select cases, will likely result in bias through the identification of atypical cases. This practice is strongly discouraged. Several types of random sampling can be used (simple random sampling, stratified, cluster). A simple random sample involves selecting cases based on a random number table for the entire caseload. An alternative method could be to identify individual clients by case manager and to then sample a certain number of cases from each grouping. Numerous survey research texts are available that explain alternative choices for sampling records and cases. Developing an appropriate sampling strategy is likely to require technical advice not usually present within case management programs. In order to produce valid information, the audit review process requires a carefully executed sampling design so that a sufficient number of representative cases are examined.

Client Record Reporting Strategy

A second strategy used to examine case management practice involves the use of a client record reporting system. This system includes information on the time taken to implement key case management activities, such as the time between client referral and the completion of the initial assessment, and the time between assessment and service delivery. The "elapsed time" data, which is recorded by project screening and case management staff, is then compiled to track the progress of the client. Results of such a tracking system can provide useful information about program functioning. For example, in the National Channeling study (Carcagno, et al, 1986), data showed that assessments were completed within an average of nine calendar days from referral (about seven working days), although 25 percent of the sample took 10 days or longer to be assessed (see Table 6-2).

Examination of the information on elapsed time from the Channeling study indicates that variation did exist across the 10 sites. For example, the Rensselaer, New York, site completed assessments in 5.7 days, while the Greater Lynn, Massachusetts, site took an average of 12.9 days. This type of comparison can also be made across case managers within a single program, or across local providers within a state program. Interpretations of these comparisons, however, must be made cautiously. Variation could have several sources: the type of clientele served by a particular case manager or project, the location or geographic area served, and/or the staffing patterns of a program. For example, a program serving a large, dispersed geographic area may be unable to complete assessments as rapidly as a more centralized site. Likewise, case managers serving a more impaired population may not be able to complete assessments quickly; disabled clients may be more difficult to schedule and may require more than one assessment home visit due to fatigue. While this information can be useful to the case management program, it must be interpreted carefully. Measures of elapsed time on various case management tasks can provide useful information for assessing program efficiency. For example, if the elapsed time between referral and assessment is

TABLE 6-2 Elapsed Time Between Client Assignment and Completion of Assessment for National Channeling Demonstration Sites by Model (in Days)

| Project | February, 1982 through September, 1983 | | |
	Mean	Median	N
Basic Case Management			
Baltimore	9.5	8.0	474
Eastern Kentucky	8.5	6.0	325
Houston	6.2	6.0	513
Middlesex County	8.3	7.0	567
Southern Maine	8.7	6.0	333
Subtotal	8.1	6.0	2,212
Financial Control			
Cleveland	10.4	7.0	593
Greater Lynn	12.9	8.0	442
Miami	12.2	10.0	652
Philadelphia	8.3	7.0	785
Rensselaer County	5.7	4.0	283
Subtotal	10.1	7.0	2,755
Total all projects	9.3	7.0	4,967

Source. Carcagno, G. J., et al. *The Evaluation of the National Long-Term Care Demonstration: The Planning and Operational Experience of the Channeling Projects.* Princeton, NJ: Mathematica Policy Research, July, 1986.

15 to 20 days, program staff may be concerned that they are not being responsive to referrals demanding prompt attention, such as those from a hospital.

This approach can also provide an indicator of whether the case management staff is completing the program forms and instruments. This indicator, however, requires careful examination. The mere fact that a form is completed does not by itself provide an indication of quality. Thorough and complete documentation is a quality indicator. Poorly implemented, however, this kind of monitoring mechanism could have negative consequences. It might inappropriately signal to case managers that the number of assessments they complete is the most important measure of their activity. Use of multiple descriptive/ process indicators will provide a broader view of program operations than reliance on a single measure.

Formalized Qualitative Review

Another method that can be applied to the client assessment process involves formalized qualitative review. In this approach, a set of standard review criteria is specified and applied to the client assessment process. An individual reviewer or review teams (depending on program size) directly observe and rate the assessment process for a random sample of cases. Review teams can be either internal staff or external reviewers, depending on program needs and circumstances. In the Channeling Demonstration, for example, independent review teams were used to perform quality control assessments, since it was necessary to ensure standardization across the 10 demonstration sites. This approach can also be used on a statewide or regional basis where multiple programs are involved. Often a modified version of the qualitative review process is used by supervisors during training. This approach involves a systematic review implemented at specified time periods, providing supervisory personnel a direct opportunity to monitor the quality of the information collected during the assessment process. Actual observation of the assessment interview provides insights into the assessment process that are not available when reviewing records. Reviewers can also immediately examine both the accuracy of the recorded information and the case managers' ability to probe and focus on an important problem. Reviewers can directly observe whether client problems (e.g. health or functional impairments, mental health difficulties, and social functioning problems) are indeed addressed in the assessment. Record review alone does not provide adequate information for supervisory personnel to determine if any specific client problems are not being identified in the assessment.

Direct observation also has limitations. First, this process is labor intensive, since both case managers and review personnel are required to be present at the assessment interview. The increased supervisory time needed for this activity may result in shortages elsewhere. Second, interviews conducted with a reviewer or supervisor present may be different than those conducted when only the case manager is present. Case managers may modify their behavior because of the presence of a reviewer. Case managers are also likely to experience heightened anxiety when accompanied by an outside reviewer, and their performance is likely to be affected. Clients may also act differently when there is an additional person present during the interview process. Despite these limitations, formalized qualitative review has some important supervisory payoffs and is recommended as a review and training device.

TO WHAT EXTENT DO THE SERVICE PLANS MEET CLIENTS' NEEDS?

Care planning is a resource allocation process in which case managers' authority and knowledge of community resources are critical.

At present, however, little is known about how best to assess whether a case manager has designed and implemented an adequate care plan. There are several strategies that can be used to examine care planning, such as:

- an audit approach
- a case review system.

Audit

The first issue is whether a formalized care plan has, in fact, been completed for each client in a timely fashion. This question can be addressed through the audit and elapsed time approaches discussed earlier. In the Channeling Demonstration, the elapsed time data source was used to record the time between the completion of an assessment and when the care plan was agreed upon by the client (the demonstration required that the client indicate approval by "signing off" on the care plan). The "elapsed" time from completed assessment to care plan sign-off was approximately 22 days. This was longer than anticipated by program planners and site administrative staff. In the Channeling intervention, the long elapsed time was re-lated to several demonstration design features, such as:

- long and comprehensive assessment protocol
- emphasis on cost calculations
- extensive involvement with informal support persons
- provider negotiations
- client understanding and sign-off on the care plan.

Programs that case manage long-term care services are faced with a difficult challenge. In arranging a package of services, it is necessary to complete a comprehensive assessment and care planning process that takes into consideration the needs of both clients *and* caregivers. Often an acute-care crisis has been the precipitating factor for the program referral and thus the client may need immediate attention. Structuring a program with a triage function is seen as an important practice element. Elapsed time then becomes a critical issue. The point of greater importance, however, is that unless valid client infor-mation exists, a discussion of the most appropriate elapsed time in relation to client needs cannot take place.

As noted earlier, in order to examine elapsed time information, a mechanism for recording client and case manager actions is needed. In agencies that currently collect and record only limited information about their clients, this will be a large undertaking. Thus, basic information about client intake is crucial in efforts to evaluate organizational effectiveness, and some systematic method of collecting intake information is strongly recommended. As noted earlier, the elapsed time analysis is another area where a sample of cases could be used rather than recording information for the entire caseload. Regardless of the method chosen, it is important for agencies responsible for arranging community-based services to monitor the intake component of their practice.

Case Review

Once it has been satisfactorily determined that a care plan has been developed, one of the most important questions is whether care plans accurately reflect client needs. Several approaches can be used to address this question. One mechanism, used most often in ongoing programs, utilizes a case review strategy. This approach generally uses an independent review team to examine a random sample of case records, comparing the information recorded on comprehensive assessment to the formalized plan of care. Reviewers rate whether the care plans represent good professional practice based on areas such as a client's diagnosis; physical, social, and environmental characteristics; and the case manager's demonstrated knowledge of the service system. For example, assume that a client assessment indicates severe cognitive impairment as evidenced by a high number of incorrect responses on one of the mental status questionnaires and reports from family members and provider personnel. On review of the care plan, however, panel members note that the plan does not include services that adequately address this particular problem. Reviewers can then raise questions about why the cognitive functioning problem was not addressed in an appropriate manner based on the client's demonstrated needs. This approach is applied to the crucial relationship between assessment data and care plan services.

An example of this type of approach was used in a recently completed review of Ohio's 2176 Waiver Program (Applebaum, Austin, & Atchley, 1987). To assess case management activities, a 3-person review team comprised of a nurse and two social workers was assembled. The panel initially developed a series of practice standards for case management and then randomly selected for review 32 clients who had been enrolled in the program for six months or longer. (This strategy was used to evaluate the care planning and monitoring procedures over time; however, a review of short-term clients may also be a beneficial monitoring activity). Following completion of the record review, in-person interviews were conducted with case managers concerning the specific cases reviewed.

Results of the review found that, in general, case managers were providing good care; however, several practice issues were raised by the team. For example, the review team found that in some instances case managers were not seeking evaluations of conditions that were potentially treatable. These included such areas as incontinence, confusion, vision and hearing problems, and polypharmacy. The panel suggested that in the absence of clinical standards to guide intervention, case managers can become less sensitive to these types of client problems. To this end, the panel recommended that case management practice standards be developed in order to increase case managers' awareness and responsiveness to potentially treatable conditions.

There are several key requirements of this type of approach. First, adequate documentation of assessment and care planning processes must be an established part of agency operations. Second, the sample of cases to be reviewed must be random and of sufficient size to ensure that the appropriate conclusions can be drawn. Third, a review panel must be established that will independently review cases. The panel should function impartially and independent of normal supervisory activities. Depending on contextual variables such as agency size, budget, and availability of outside expertise, the review panel may be either internal or external, with the major criterion for selection being an understanding of long-term care clients and the systems. An external review panel has an advantage of autonomy as well as providing fresh perspectives to the organization. Its disadvantages are that it may be costly and time-consuming. In addition, recruiting a panel that could be available on an ongoing basis may be difficult. Some agencies have used both internal *and* external reviewers in an effort to gain the advantages of having external review while reducing some of the costs by having external reviews completed less frequently.

A case review process provides case managers with an independent feedback mechanism for their care planning. Since designing a plan of care requires both creativity and attention to detail, the opportunity to receive feedback on care plans can be very valuable. Such a process can serve as both a quality assurance mechanism and as a supervisory activity. The major disadvantage of the case review process is that it is based on a paper review without direct contact with clients. It is often difficult for reviewers who only have access to forms to appreciate the complex circumstances surrounding care plan development. Inadequate documentation concerning care (which many argue is a practice problem) can be easily interpreted as poor practice when in reality it may reflect good care, but poor records. A second problem involves the subjectivity of care planning in long-term care. In many cases, a client problem can be addressed through several different mechanisms, all of which meet professional practice standards. Professional reviewers are often unable to agree on the one "best practice" approach to a plan of care. This suggests that a review panel should include professionals with different perspectives. It is also necessary that program staff recognize the diversity in case management practice and the need to agree on a clear set of practice standards.

A second example of this method was a care plan research project conducted by Temple University as part of the Channeling Demonstration (Schneider, Hirsh, Rikards, Sterthous, Cohen, & Wilson, 1986). The study examined a sample of client records from each of the 10 Channeling sites, comparing the type and number of problems on each client's baseline assessment to the initial care plan. The methodology involved classifying problems into specific categories and then comparing whether the assessment problems were addressed in the structured care plan.

One particularly interesting finding was that, despite only minor differences in the characteristics of clients on the number and type of problems identified at assessment, some major differences existed in the problems addressed in the formalized care plans. Care plans of case managers in the five Channeling sites that had more resources available for purchasing community services (known as financial control model channeling) differed from the care plans of case managers in the sites that provided a limited amount of funds for client services (basic Channeling). Case managers working with more limited resources (in the basic sites) addressed problems involving medical care, financial resources, informal supports, social activities, housing problems, and legal problems, while case managers with more resources (the financial control sites) identified more problems with personal care and emotional and health problems. The Temple University researchers hypothesized that access to services and purchasing power may have influenced the type of problems identified by case managers in the two Channeling models.

This research suggests that developing a care plan, while based on characteristics of clients and their environment, also includes a subjective component. In the Temple study, case manager identification of client problems was apparently influenced by their recognition that they could, in fact, resolve these problems. Case managers in the basic model (a brokering model) focused on problems that could be solved within the resource constraints of their position. However, case managers with control over resources (service management) focused on the direct personal care needs of clients rather than on the broader base of services addressed by the basic model case managers. In developing case management systems, understanding how resource availability can affect case manager behavior is critical to program designers. Although there is much more to learn about the tasks of a case manager, it is clear that structural elements such as control over resources significantly affects case management practice.

Attempting to determine whether a care plan accurately reflects the needs of an individual client is difficult at best. Research has shown that even the most highly qualified professionals using the same client information may not agree on what constitutes the best care plan. Several studies (Schneider, et al., 1986; Sager, 1977) have reported this finding. Thus, evaluating this component of case management remains an important but challenging area for case managers, program administrators, and evaluators.

A final care planning issue is the degree to which services in care plans are designed with cost in mind. As noted earlier, today's case managers face dual responsibilities and function both as service arrangers for clients and as gatekeepers for the service system. Once a client is determined to be eligible for the community-based long-term care system, the case manager more and more often has to ensure that the service plan is developed within some specific cost limits. Monitoring this aspect of case management practice is an important organizational responsibility. Normal supervisory review of the care plans and use of independent review teams as previously discussed can be helpful here. Service management or managed-care case management programs with control over service expenditures, such as the five Financial Control Channeling sites, or projects operating under the home and community-based waiver authority (2176) or the On Lok and Social/HMO projects, have established information and financial tracking systems that perform this review function. For instance, in the Channeling Demonstration, each financial control site had an automated management information system that included the cost of the care plan for each client enrolled. In addition to monitoring costs for each individual client, the average cost of each case manager's caseload was also examined (see Table 6–3). These data provided additional monitoring capacity for examining service expenditures. Supervisors could examine patterns of services and costs of care plans across case managers. It was possible to observe that a particular worker was spending an average $600 per month on client services, while the average for the agency was $400, indicating the need for more in-depth supervisory review. In the Social/HMO sites, initial care plans are presented at case conferences where comprehen-

TABLE 6-3 Care Plan Budget Control Report Table*
Summary Totals

Case manager	Number of clients			Estimated care plan cost	Estimated % of SNF/ICF level
	Active	Inactive	Total		
1	35	3	38	$381.64	27.26%
2	32	7	39	391.30	27.95
3	45	1	46	377.44	26.96
4	43	1	44	391.16	27.94
5	34	8	42	425.88	30.42
6	35	4	39	433.16	30.94
7	38	1	39	458.78	32.77
8	37	1	38	410.90	29.35
9	44	1	45	452.20	32.3
10	31	10	41	477.40	34.1
Agency Totals	374	37	411	419.98	29.99

*Summary information from the Care Plan Budget Control Report.
**From the Client Status Column of the report (manual totaling).

Source. Carcagno, G.J., et al. *The Evaluation of the National Long-Term Care Demonstration: The Planning and Operational Experience of the Channeling Projects.* Princeton, NJ: Mathematica Policy Research, July, 1986.

siveness and quality as well as costs are discussed. In addition, the Social/HMO projects monitor costs of care plans for enrollees who are "in benefit" closely to determine ongoing appropriateness of care plans and potential substitution of services (Leutz, et al., 1985).

ARE THE SERVICE PLANS DESIGNED ACTUALLY IMPLEMENTED?

Because the care plan is just that—a plan—examining whether the services are delivered as designed is an essential component of evaluative activities. Ensuring that clients do, in fact, receive the services specified in the care plan is a key case management function. However, mere receipt of services is not enough. While community-based care is an attractive choice for many persons, it is also difficult to monitor the quality of care provided.

To some extent, approaches to assessing the quality of ongoing services are dependent on the type of case management model being implemented. For example, direct provider monitoring practices are possible where case management agencies have budget control over a wide range of services and actually authorize the purchase of services from providers who are *generally* under contract (the service management models). However, agencies using the broker model without controls on service dollars, are more limited in the type and extent of monitoring activities they can impose on providers.

The Channeling Demonstration provides a good example of this distinction. In five of the sites where project case managers had only limited funds to purchase community services for long-term care clients (the Basic model), the vast majority of services provided to Channeling clients were funded by other sources. Under these circumstances, demonstration personnel did not feel that they could require service providers to inform case managers about service provision, and they could not mandate provider contact at specified time periods. As a result, two monitoring approaches with minimal service provider involvement were developed. First, client contact logs were kept in which case managers recorded contacts with clients, family members, informal supports, and formal service providers. The logs were used to document initial service delivery. For example, within seven days following the ordering of a new service, case managers were to contact both the client and the service provider to verify delivery. A systematic review of case manager logs in conjunction with other program records provided documentation for provider monitoring activities. Although this approach can document that service delivery did in fact occur, it does not provide information about timeliness of services delivery or about service quality.

In order to supplement this approach, two of the Channeling sites used staff members other than the primary case manager to perform a follow up assessment. During reassessment, this staff member examined how well the initial care plan had been implemented. A formalized system of reviewing care plans could be developed as part of this follow-up assessment process. For example, a form could be used in which reassessors examine initial care plan objectives and services ordered and compare them to current needs and services.

This approach is not, however, without limitations. Most importantly, the proposal to have a different staff person conduct reassessments may be troublesome to both case managers and clients. Case managers and clients often develop close relationships, and this approach can be disruptive to the continuity of these relationships. An additional problem is that changes in a client's condition may be difficult to interpret, such that the process may not provide useful information to help improve case management practice. Reports from agencies using this approach are somewhat mixed. Some agencies report that such a mechanism provided useful feedback to case managers, while others have indicated that the problems caused by the lack of continuity did not outweigh the benefits. As with each of the approaches discussed in this section, case management staff have to examine their needs and objectives in determining which activities warrant further exploration.

In contrast, the five sites of the Channeling Demonstration that had considerable control over community-based service dollars (the financial control model) used other provider monitoring approaches. Although still relying on contacts with clients, informal caregivers, and providers, more formalized procedures were also developed. As part of their contractual obligations, service providers were required to call case managers after the initial service visit. A systematic recording and review of calls provided important data on provider performance. In select sites, in-home service providers were contractually required to complete brief monthly reports on the clients' conditions and services received. This type of monitoring also improved care by keeping case managers aware of client conditions and circumstances. The experience of the Channeling Demonstration illustrates that systematic monitoring of provider performance can be incorporated into the contracting process as well.

It is important to emphasize that efforts to ensure effectiveness of the services arranged for clients by the case management agency require strong commitment on the part of the organization. Experience with the provision of case management indicates that organizations rely almost exclusively on case managers to monitor the quality of care provided by contracted service providers. However, quality assurance should also be the responsibility of the agency, rather than solely the responsibility of case management staff. Case managers play an integral role in ensuring quality, but their roles and responsibilities need to be part of an overall quality assurance system.

ARE CLIENTS SATISFIED WITH THE CASE-MANAGED CARE RECEIVED?

Client satisfaction with the care received as a result of the case management intervention is an area of considerable interest. This topic has been examined in a number of ways including client surveys, participation rate analysis, and termination rate analysis.

The survey approach is a direct method in which clients are asked about case management activities and services received. Although this does not involve a comparison with another client group, it provides important descriptive information and serves as an indication of how clients feel about case management and services received. For example, if low satisfaction is consistently reported, this might suggest a particular problem area to be investigated.

One example of this approach was used in a recent survey of caregivers in Ohio's long-term care case management program (Applebaum, Austin, & Atchley, 1987). In this study, 50 caregivers were randomly selected and asked questions concerning the quality of the program and the difficulties they faced in providing care to program clients. Caregivers, who were interviewed by telephone, reported high satisfaction with the program (88% very satisfied or satisfied) although they also reported several stressful aspects of the caregiving role. Information from the survey provided some insights to the organization about the needs of caregivers and also an indication that the program was helping caregivers in their efforts to provide care.

The major disadvantage of this survey approach is that results are difficult to interpret. Since there is no comparison group, it is difficult to know whether the results represent a valid indicator of good case management. An example from the evaluation of the Channeling Demonstration illustrates this point. In Channeling, program clients were asked about their satisfaction with current service arrangements. A review of the results for program clients (see Table 6–4) showed that just over 93 percent of the clients were satisfied or partly satisfied with service arrangements. Based on these results, program staff might have concluded that they were doing a good job of providing services. However, when data are examined for individuals in the demonstration's control group (those who did not receive program services), a slightly different conclusion is suggested. Data in Table 6–4 show that a fairly comparable number (almost 92%) of the control group reported being satisfied or partly satisfied with service arrangements. This example underscores the importance of having a comparison group when attempting to interpret client reports regarding outcomes such as satisfaction.

In addition to this major problem there are a series of other barriers to conducting good evaluation research including the development of valid and reliable measures, adequate sample size, and sound data collection techniques. For example, rigorous collection of survey data can be costly and time consuming; professional interviews can easily cost $25 to $30 per client. If programs try to cut costs by having case managers collect survey information, significant reporting bias can be introduced. Clients may be hesitant to complain about a particular case manager or service for fear of jeopardizing the care they are receiving. Thus, while the survey process is a common mode of data collection, it has several significant limitations.

The other approaches to examining client satisfaction analyze information on participation and termination rates. For example, in the Channeling Demonstration, data were kept on the number of clients

TABLE 6–4 Impacts on Satisfaction With Service Arrangement (Percent)

	Six months		
	Treatment group mean	Control group mean	Treatment/ control difference
Satisfaction with service arrangement			
Satisfied	73.6%	72.1%	1.5%
Partly satisfied	19.6	19.4	.1
Dissatisfied	6.9	8.6	−1.7
Sample size	1,031	558	1,589

The differences in the above data are not statistically significant when analyzed using the following tests:
• Different from zero statistically at the 5 percent significance level, using a two-tailed test.
• Different from zero statistically at the 1 percent significance level, using a two-tailed test.

Source: Applebaum, R., Harrigan, M. *Channeling Effects on the Quality of Clients' Lives*. Princeton, NJ: Mathematica Policy Research, April, 1986.

who were determined to be eligible, but who then did not receive services. The refusal rate was approximately 10 percent (see Table 6–5). If a program's rate was substantially higher than that, it might serve as an indicator that clients did not perceive that their needs were being met by the program. For example, a cumbersome and long assessment process, resulting in a high refusal rate, might suggest that a program should streamline the assessment process.

Similarly, rates of termination, those clients who enter and then withdraw, could also provide useful information on program operations. In the Channeling Demonstration, about 50 percent of the clients were no longer enrolled in the demonstration 12 months after entry (see Table 6–6). In this case, just over 40 percent of the demonstration clients had either died or had gone into nursing homes. However, had this number been comprised largely of clients refusing care or withdrawing from the project, that might have been an indicator of lower client satisfaction. Once again, this kind of information can contribute to an understanding of program operations, although it is not a definitive measure of program effectiveness.

The strategies examined in this chapter represent a sample of the types of quality assurance activities that could be undertaken by a case management agency. Each case management program needs to examine its specific needs, wants, and resources in order to deter-

TABLE 6–5 Clients Terminated 12 Months After Assignment to Channeling, by Reason and Time Period

Item	Between random assignment and assessment	Between assessment and completion of care plan	After completion of care plan and service initiation	Total
Clients assigned				2,108
Clients terminated	231	225	679	1,135
Percent	11.0%	10.7%	32.2%	53.8%
Reason for termination (Percent)				
Died	1.7	2.7	14.0	18.4
Institutionalized	0.6	2.0	9.4	12.0
Refused	7.8	2.8	3.7	14.2
Insufficient disability	0.1	2.2	0.8	3.1
Moved/unable to locate	0.4	0.4	2.4	3.2
Condition stabilized	0.0	0.1	1.7	1.8
Too service-dependent	0.0	0.3	0.2	0.6
Refused cost sharing	—	—	—	—
Not Medicare-eligible	—	—	—	—
Other	0.4	0.1	0.0	0.6

Source Carcagno, G.J., et al. *The Evaluation of the National Long-Term Care Demonstration: The Planning and Operational Experience of the Channeling Projects.* Princeton, NJ: Mathematica Policy Research, July, 1986.

mine which types of activities make sense for the organization. The range of quality assurance activities and the evaluative needs of the agency must be clearly understood. In the next chapter, approaches to evaluating the impact of case management will be presented.

TABLE 6–6 Percent Active by Month (12-Month Cohort) for First 12 Months Treatments Enrolled in Channeling

Project	Sample	Month											
		1	2	3	4	5	6	7	8	9	10	11	12
Basic case management													
Baltimore	484	78.7	74.0	67.8	65.9	62.9	59.1	56.2	53.7	51.9	49.6	46.9	44.4
Eastern Kentucky	294	88.8	83.3	79.6	74.5	71.1	69.0	67.3	65.3	63.3	60.9	59.5	57.8
Houston	472	83.1	78.0	73.7	68.4	63.8	59.5	57.2	55.5	54.0	51.9	49.2	47.7
Middlesex County	528	83.0	75.0	69.1	62.9	57.2	53.6	50.8	48.7	45.1	41.7	39.6	37.9
Southern Maine	330	81.5	74.2	67.6	66.7	63.6	60.3	57.3	55.8	53.9	51.8	50.9	49.4
Total	2,108	82.6	76.5	71.1	67.0	62.9	59.4	56.8	54.8	52.6	50.0	48.0	46.2
Financial Control													
Cleveland	506	90.9	79.8	74.3	69.6	66.8	64.4	60.7	59.3	56.5	54.0	51.2	49.8
Greater Lynn	391	85.9	76.0	69.8	65.7	62.4	59.3	57.5	55.0	52.4	49.4	48.8	48.3
Miami	597	80.4	72.7	68.0	63.8	61.3	60.6	57.6	56.3	54.8	52.6	51.1	49.4
Philadelphia	774	86.6	79.8	75.6	70.9	67.1	64.2	62.1	60.5	57.9	56.3	54.4	52.6
Rensselaer County	230	84.3	79.1	74.3	69.6	68.3	63.9	60.9	58.7	57.0	54.3	52.6	51.3
Total	2,498	85.7	77.5	72.5	68.0	65.0	62.6	59.9	58.2	55.9	53.7	51.9	50.5
All projects	4,606	84.3	77.0	71.8	67.6	64.0	61.1	58.5	56.6	54.4	52.0	50.1	48.5

Source. Carcagno, G.J., et al. *The Evaluation of the National Long-Term Care Demonstration: The Planning and Operational Experience of the Channeling Projects.* Princeton, NJ: Mathematica Policy Research, July, 1986.

Chapter **7**

Assessing the Outcomes of Case Management Practice

The quality assurance or descriptive evaluation approaches that have been discussed to this point have focused on descriptive and process indicators. In this chapter, methods for studying the outcomes or impact of case managed services on program clients are presented. The key difference between this approach and the approach described in the previous chapter involves the use of a comparative design.

COMPARATIVE OUTCOMES APPROACH

The major question in a comparative approach is: Does the case management intervention result in benefits for those receiving such care compared to a nonprogram client group with similar characteristics?

In this approach, evaluators always ask whether the client group receiving program services had different outcomes when compared to a nonprogram client group with similar characteristics. This question, addressed in over 15 federal and state demonstrations over the last 15 years, has received considerable attention (Kemper et al., 1987). The studies undertaken to address this question vary in their methodological approaches, but all have attempted to compare case-managed community-based long-term care with the traditional long-term care system.

Client Level Outcomes   **Service Utilization Outcomes**

Physical functioning   Nursing home use (admissions, days)

Mortality   Hospital use (admissions, days)

Mental status   Community service use

Life quality   Total costs of care

Social functioning

Unmet needs

The design of comparative studies is affected by the nature of the group being evaluated. In some cases the unit of analysis might be a relatively small group; in other instances an entire county or region might be the unit of analysis. The nature of the group to be evaluated will clearly influence the evaluation design. Several comparative evaluation designs are examined below.

Counties

One approach to evaluating projects providing countywide intervention involves using comparison counties. For example, the ACCESS Project in New York (Price and Ripp, 1980) used this strategy. Researchers in that project selected six counties from throughout New York State that they felt most closely resembled the demographic and service characteristics of the county that ACCESS served. Pre- and postmeasures in several areas of public health and long-term care costs, for example, were examined for the six comparison counties and the intervention county. In this study, nursing home costs under Medicaid in the intervention county were found to have increased at a significantly lower rate than in the comparison counties.

Proponents of this technique suggest that, if the evaluation objective is to test a system-level intervention, this is the only design that will provide the necessary data. Critics of this design identify the major drawback as the difficulty in identifying appropriate comparison counties. It is extremely difficult to ensure that comparison counties are indeed comparable because of regional variations in demographic characteristics and long-term care systems (both institutional and noninstitutional). Thus, evaluations using this strategy must contend with criticisms concerning the degree of comparability. It is important to note that in this approach data are compared at an aggregate level (i.e., county). Client specific information is not examined. In other studies, comparisons to individuals residing in other counties have been undertaken. This approach is discussed in the following section.

This type of design, despite some of the limitations just discussed, may be particularly relevant when an intervention is being tested in a well-defined area of a state or region. For example, many programs are currently testing Medicaid waivers for home and community-based care through Section 2176 of the 1981 Budget Reconciliation Act by implementing case management in selected parts of their states. Under these circumstances where an entire county is being tested, a model that compares countywide data on selected outcome variables may be a feasible evaluation design. Careful selection of comparison counties or regions and measures examined is, however, extremely important in a study of this nature.

Program and Nonprogram Participants

A second approach (which is the dominant methodology used in previous community care demonstrations) involves comparing a group of program participants to a group of nonprogram clients with similar characteristics. The evaluation principle behind this method is that the only difference that should exist between program and nonprogram groups is a result of receiving the case management intervention. To ensure comparability, two design approaches have been used. One uses a random assignment methodology in which individuals are randomly assigned to receive either case-managed care or to receive the long-term care services normally available in the community. The second approach uses a matched comparison group.

The strength of a randomized approach is that, with careful research procedures and sample size, researchers can be confident that the two groups being studied are equivalent, thus yielding more confidence in the results. Eight previous community-based long-term care demonstrations including the Channeling Demonstration used a randomized research design. In the Channeling Demonstration, individuals were screened by the intake units in each of the 10 program sites. Those individuals passing the screen and interested in participating in the research demonstration were then randomly assigned to either receive project services or to receive the care normally available in the community. Researchers used a computerized system to randomly assign group status to individuals as they passed the screen. Careful procedures had to be designed to guard against administrative problems such as procedures for individuals reapplying after receiving a group assignment.

Although the principles of randomized design are generally straightforward, implementing the technique can be much more difficult. Service providers are often reluctant to become involved with a program that they perceive as arbitrarily withholding needed services from individuals in the nonprogram group. This can result in resistance both from within the agency and also from referral sources and providers. Providers are concerned with the ethical issues surrounding this type of intervention. It is our contention that in circumstances in which a particular intervention has not been subject to evaluation techniques, testing that intervention is, in fact, ethical practice. In addition to the political and ethical aspects of this type of experimental design, a multitude of design problems often arise during implementation. Because of the importance of ensuring the integrity of a randomized design, it is recommended that projects use outside consultation in deciding when and how to use this type of experimental design.

Results from recent demonstrations provide a sample of the type of comparisons that can be made in an evaluative design of this nature. For example, in Table 7–1, data on the use of nursing homes show that after 12 months, program clients in the Channeling Demonstration spent about 17 days on average in a nursing home compared to just over 20 days for control group members. In this case, the differences are relatively small and not statistically significant (which means 95 percent of the time, differences of this size would indicate that there are no actual differences between groups). In a similar type of study conducted in South Carolina, program and nonprogram group differences were of a much larger magnitude. Program clients had on average 40 fewer days of nursing home use than nonprogram group members. Although one of these studies (South Carolina) showed program effects and the other (Channeling) did not, the major point is that, without the ability to compare pro-

TABLE 7–1 Nursing Home Use in Two Select Community Care
Evaluations After 12 Months

| | Number of days in nursing home (at 12 months) | | |
Evaluation	Treatment group mean	Control group mean	Treatment/control difference
Channeling Demonstration	17.0	20.2	−3.2
South Carolina Community Care Demonstration	90	130	−40*

*Statistically different from zero at the five percent level, using a two-tailed test.

Source. Applebaum, R., Harrigan, M., Kemper, P. *The Evaluation of the National Long-Term Care Demonstration: Tables Comparing Channeling to Other Community Care Demonstrations*. Princeton, NJ: Mathematica Policy Research, May, 1986.

gram results to the experience of a comparison group, it is not possible to conclude that effects have occurred as a result of the program.

A second approach used to ensure group comparability is to use a matched comparison group. Several techniques for matching have been used in earlier long-term care studies (Birnbaum, et al., 1985; Zawadski, et al., 1984; Miller, et al., 1984; and Shealy, Hicks, & Quinn, 1979). Evaluators generally attempt to recruit comparison group members in the same way that the program recruits applicants. The advantage of this approach is that it provides the evaluation with a comparison group without going through the difficulties often associated with using a randomized design. Its major disadvantage, however, is that it is often difficult to simulate the program recruiting process and thus difficult to ensure that the comparison group is indeed comparable.

The On Lok Demonstration conducted in San Francisco's Chinatown illustrates the difficulty of such a design. Because On Lok served all of Chinatown, it had to go outside of the area to recruit comparison group members. This proved to be a problem, since it was difficult in other areas to recruit individuals with similar characteristics. Thus, although the project was able to recruit a comparison group, it could not say with confidence that the groups were comparable, and this weakened the evaluation findings. The difficulty of ensuring comparability is thus the Achilles' heel of comparison group evaluative approaches. Implementing a matched research design presents important challenges, and agencies should expect that consultation will be required. However, because comparison group design does not require randomly assigning applicants, it remains an appealing option in many cases.

One important principle must be reemphasized here regarding the use of this type of evaluation design. *Having a comparison group that closely resembles the program client population is essential to study success; therefore, procedures used to make group assignments are critical.* Studies using this design must identify comparison group members, to the extent possible, in the same manner in which program clients are recruited or enter the program. This is no easy task and, in fact, the "easy" solution to recruiting a comparison group does not work in most instances. For example, a commonly used recruiting method has been to take individuals who have been rejected from the program and ask them to participate in the research as comparison group members. Because these individuals often are different from those accepted into the program (for example, more or less disabled, have higher income), these individuals may fare better or worse than program clients, differences that may not necessarily be related to the program interventions. Thus, case management programs electing to use this approach must carefully examine their methods for creating the comparison group. Keep in mind that a poorly designed study may be worse than no study at all.

Agency Evaluative Options

Given the difficulties associated with using a matched comparison methodology and the limited circumstances in which a randomized design is appropriate, what choices exist for program personnel interested in evaluating program outcomes?

Unfortunately, there are no easy answers to this question. One potential strategy involves testing of a new program design compared to the existing intervention. This model, used in programs that are interested in testing a variation of their current practice, is relatively straightforward. Rather than implementing a totally new intervention—because they believe it is an improvement over current practice—a comparative evaluation is designed in which the traditional and alternative interventions can be compared. For example, one study of this nature, conducted by the ACCESS project examined a more in-depth case management approach compared to their existing model of case management practice (Eggert, et al., 1986). This study randomly assigned applicants to one of two case management approaches. One model used the traditional ACCESS case management approach for monitoring direct services, but without direct service provision, while the other used a case management and service worker team method to both provide services and case management. Results of the study showed that the clients under the new case management approach used fewer health and long-term care services than clients under the traditional model, with no reported differences in life quality.

Although the results of this particular study need further examination, they are important for several reasons. First, it should be noted that this study was done by an agency that was one of the first organizations in the country to provide long-term care case management. Their approach to case management had been well established, and the fact that they were willing to test an alternative approach provides a useful example to other agencies. Continually testing new strategies and approaches is an important concept for human service agencies to recognize. A second point involves the research approach used in this study. By using a viable research design this study was able to test a new intervention with some confidence, thus providing a model for programs interested in evaluating a new intervention.

The more traditional randomized experimental design has also been used in some ongoing programs, particularly those that receive applications from more clients than can be served by the organization. Under these circumstances, different models of experimental design might be feasible. In general, however, once an intervention has been adopted in mainstream practice—whether it be the polio vaccine, fluoride in the water, or case management—a pure experimental approach in which applicants are randomly assigned is no longer feasible.

In summary, program impact cannot be assessed without the use of some type of comparison methodology. Unless the experiences of those receiving services can be compared to those not receiving such care, either at the individual or county level, then program impacts cannot be directly ascertained. Unfortunately, the most rigorous experimental design used to determine program outcomes, the randomized research design, is often very difficult to implement, particularly in an ongoing program. Although program personnel want to present outcome data on major program functions, it is frequently difficult to design an evaluation that is both rigorous and politically feasible. Thus, it is necessary to develop a broad based strategy that combines quality assurance and evaluation activities in a systematic manner. Carefully planning this evaluative strategy is a major challenge faced by all case management agencies.

Part III

PAST EXPERIENCES AND FUTURE CHALLENGES

"Those who cannot remember the past are condemned to repeat it." SANTAYANA

"The trouble with our times is that the future is not what it used to be." PAUL VALÉRY

"There is a simple solution to everything, neat, feasible, and wrong." H. L. MENCKEN

Chapter **8**

The Evolution of Case Management Service Delivery

Case management has been provided by a number of different programs and organizations. This chapter reviews service delivery experiences in the provision of case management services in a range of settings including: long-term care demonstration projects, Area Agencies on Aging, the Medicaid Home and Community-Based Waiver Program, the Robert Wood Johnson Hospital Initiatives in Long-Term Care Projects, and case management that is being incorporated in some private long-term care insurance plans. The evolution of case management in these settings is discussed in the sections that follow.

LONG-TERM CARE DEMONSTRATIONS

Over the past 16 years, long-term care demonstrations have been funded to develop community-based long-term care delivery systems and services. Medicare (Section 222 of the Social Security Amendments of 1972, PL 92-603) and Medicaid (Section 115 of PL 92-603) waivers have permitted more flexible eligibility and fewer restrictions on the range of services offered. Table 8–1 presents information on 18 demonstration projects. Each project incorporated two common elements: coverage of an expanded array of community-based services, and case management. The types and comprehensiveness of services

TABLE 8–1 Delivery System Characteristics of Long-Term Care Projects

Project	Organizational auspices	Targeting	Gatekeeping	Financing/ Reimbursement
ON Lok III 4/71 start 1983–present Phase III	independent, private nonprofit provider agency	• 55+ • Medicare eligible • 10% Medicaid • ICF/SNF certified	• prior authorization of waivered services • centralized authorization power	• Medicare waiver • prospective reimbursement • provider risk • capitated funding
Wisconsin CCO 8/73–12/79	2 independent, private, nonprofit 1 county public agency 1 provider 2 nonprovider	• 65+ • at risk of nursing home placement • functionally impaired • potential for discharge from nursing home • about to be discharged from hospital • need for community services • monitoring & education needed	• prior authorization of waivered services	• Medicaid • retrospective reimbursement • some private pay clients accepted
Triage 2/74–3/79	freestanding case management agency (private nonprofit)	• 65+ Medicare eligible	• prior authorization of waivered services	• Medicare • retrospective reimbursement
WA Community based care 7/75–7/79	specially created state government agencies (2 sites)	• 18+ • Medicaid eligible • at risk of nursing home placement	• prior authorization of waivered services	• Medicare & Medicaid • retrospective reimbursement

Program	Organization	Client Eligibility	Authorization	Reimbursement
		• funcitonally impaired • potential for discharge from nursing home • about to be discharged from hospital	• prior authorization of waivered services	• Medicare & Medicaid • retrospective reimbursement • 75% cap on individual budget • available to private pay clients
ACCESS 7/75–present	freestanding case management agency (private nonprofit)	• 18+ • ICF/SNF certified • preadmission screening • at risk of nursing home placement • functionally impaired • mental functioning problems • under care plan cost limit • potential for discharge from nursing home • about to be discharged from hospital		
Georgia's AHS 7/76–3/81	existing government provider agency	• 50+ • medicaid eligible • ICF/SNF certified • at risk of nursing home placement • funcitonally impaired	• prior authorization of waivered services • 85% cap on individual budgets	• Medicaid • retrospective reimbursement • 85% cap on individual budgets

125

TABLE 8–1 (Continued)

Project	Organizational auspices	Targeting	Gatekeeping	Financing/Reimbursement
PROJECT OPEN 9/78–6/83	Hospital & consortium of community social service provider agency	• 65+ • Medical eligible • at risk of nursing home placement • functionally impaired • recently hospitalized • at risk of frequent hospital admissions • monitoring and education needed	• prior authorization of waivered services	• Medicare • prospective reimbursement
San Diego LTCP 3/79–1/84	home health care provider agency	• 65+ • Medical eligible • at risk of nursing home placement • functionally impaired • recently hospitalized • at risk of frequent hospital admissions • monitoring and education needed	• prior authorization of waivered services	• Medicare • retrospective reimbursement
Oregon Fig-Waiver 7/79–6/81	implemented in ongoing provider agencies. No management agency	• 65+ • Medicaid eligible • potential for discharge from nursing home	• prior authorization of waivered services • 75% cap on individual budgets	• Medicaid, Administration on Aging Model projects grant, and state funds

		• about to be discharged from hospital		• retrospective reimbursement • 75% cap on individual budgets • Medicaid • retrospective reimbursement • 75% cap on individual budgets
MSSP 7/79–present	existing public and private nonprofit provider agencies	• 65+ • Medicaid • at risk of nursing home placement • mental functioning problems • under care plan cost limit • major loss or crisis • potential for discharge from nursing home • about to be discharged from hospital • recently hospitalized • at risk of frequent hospital admissions	• prior authorization of waivered services • 75% cap on individual budgets	
Texas ICF II 1/80–12/85	State government provider agency	• 18+ • Medicaid eligible • potential for discharge from nursing home • deinstitutionalization of some ICF II residents • preadmission	• prior authorization of waivered services	• Medicaid • retrospective reimbursement

TABLE 8–1 (Continued)

Project	Organizational auspices	Targeting	Gatekeeping	Financing/ Reimbursement
		screening of potential ICF II residents		
New York Nursing Home Without Walls 3/80–present	existing home care provider agencies certified as project agencies	• 18+ • Medicaid eligible • potential for discharge from nursing home • preadmission screening	• prior authorization of waivered services • 75% cap on individual budgets	• Medicaid • retrospective reimbursement • 75% cap on individual budgets • available to private pay clients
South Carolina CLTC 7/80–11/84	existing government agency (nonprovider)	• 18+ • Medicare or Medicaid eligible • ICF/SNF certified • preadmission screening • functionally impaired	• prior authorization of waivered services • 75% cap on individual budgets	• Medicare, Medicaid, Appalachia Regional Commission funds & state funds • prospective & retrospective reimbursement • 75% cap on individual budgets
New York Home Care Project 10/80–3/84	existing public and private nonprofit agencies	• 65+ • Medicare eligible • ICF/SNF certified • functionally impaired • mental functioning problems	• prior authorization of waivered services	• Medicare • prospective & retrospective reimbursement

Project / Dates	Agency	Target Population	Authorization / Controls	Funding / Reimbursement
Florida Pentastar 1/81–10/83	existing government planning agency	• 60+ • Medicaid eligible • at risk of nursing home placement	• prior authorization of waivered services	• Medicaid • retrospective reimbursement
Channeling Basic Model 2/82–3/85	4 comprehensive human service agencies 1 freestanding dept. on aging 4 are providers 1 nonprovider	• 65+ • functionally impaired • mental functioning problems • major loss or crisis • unmet needs/fragile informal support system	• prior authorization of waivered services	• each site received an award of $250,000 from DHHS to be used for service expansion & gap-filling • client cost sharing • prospective & retrospective reimbursement
Channeling Financial Control Model 2/82–3/85	2 comprehensive human service agencies 3 freestanding depts. on aging 4 are providers 1 nonprovider	• 65+ • medicare eligible • functionally impaired • mental functioning problems • under care plan cost limit • major loss or crisis • unmet needs/fragile informal support system	• prior authorization of waivered services • 85% cap on individual budgets • 60% cap on agency budget	• Medicare, Medicaid, Title II, and Social Service Block grant funds • prospective reimbursement • client cost sharing • pooled funding • 85% cap on individual budget • 60% cap on agency budget
Social/HMO 3/85	varies by site	• representative population of elderly; well, moderately impaired and frail	• long-term care plan required • service limits • nonrenewability of some parts of coverage • preadmission screening	• funding pool (Medicare, Medicaid, SSBG.) • monthly premiums • co-insurance

*In all projects, case managers were able to offer an expanded array of services, which increased their flexibility in prescribing services. What is focused on here is the way in which specific reimbursement variables affect case managers' ability to prescribe services.

available to clients of each project depended on whether a Medicare or Medicaid waiver was present and on the overall design of the demonstration. The role of case management varied considerably in different settings. The specific case management model implemented in each project was a function of the four programmatic variables examined in Chapter 3: financing, targeting, gatekeeping, and organizational auspices. The projects are presented in chronological order to observe how these basic demonstration project components have shifted over time.

Financing

The majority of demonstrations relied on Medicare and/or Medicaid waivers for financing. These waivers permitted more flexible use of Medicare and Medicaid funds to finance home- and community-based services for eligible clients. These projects were retrospectively reimbursed, with cost-based financing paid following the provision of services. ACCESS was the first project to incorporate a budget on the costs of individual care plans. The Georgia Alternative Health Services project, the Oregon FIG-Waiver, the Multiservice Senior Program, New York's Nursing Home Without Walls, the South Carolina Community Long-Term Care demonstration, and the Financial Control Model of Channeling also included this financing feature.

The Social/HMO and the Financial Control Model of Channeling also included a funds pool. In these projects, funds from a number of different sources (e.g., Medicare, Medicaid, private premiums, Title III of the Older Americans Act, and Title XX) were pooled for the entire caseload. Care plans were then developed within specific budgetary guidelines, and payment for the care plans drawn from the pooled fund without regard to the individual funding source.

On Lok III and the Social/HMO, which are still operational, were the only demonstrations prospectively reimbursed. These projects received a capitated amount for each eligible client. Here the major innovation was the introduction of provider risk. The demonstrations were at risk to meet the costs of care plans developed by case managers. If costs exceeded the aggregate capitated amount the projects incurred a loss. If costs fell below, the project created a surplus.

Over time, demonstration financing has become increasingly structured and controlled. The introduction of budget caps in conjunction with the use of preadmission screening was designed to tighten and control both targeting and the costs of care plans. Prospective financing and provider risk represent next steps in this developmental process. If providers are at risk, it can be anticipated that they will impose greater control, monitoring, and sanctions, in efforts to more carefully manage the provision of services to eligible clients. The capacity of providers to actually work within the constraints of a prospective payment system will depend in part on their confidence that case management tasks are implemented with high levels of validity and reliability. Provider risk requires agencies to systematically track and monitor the eligibility process, the development of care plans, the costs of care plans, and changes in client circumstances that might alter their care plans.

These demonstrations can be viewed as evolutionary with more recent projects incorporating a more complex case management function than earlier efforts. Emphasis on client targeting and cost controls was expanded as efforts to demonstrate cost-effectiveness became dominant. Capitman (1986), for example, identified several key elements that reflected the expanded role of case management: targeting goals, methods for identifying clients, greater control over service utilization, control of services beyond the scope of the waiver, target budgets or capitated reimbursement. "Increasingly the scope of case management and the use of other cost control mechanisms while constraining the costs of the administrative service appear to be important ingredients in design of successful community long-term care programs." (Capitman, 1986, p. 403)

Targeting

Targeting criteria in the demonstrations fell into four categories: program eligibility, age, level of impairment, and location in the delivery system.

Sixteen of the projects required either Medicare and/or Medicaid eligibility. Nine focused on the population over age 65; five included persons over age 18 and four targeted clients over age 50 or 55. Projects used a variety of methods to determine level of impairment. Ten projects used measures of "functional impairment" by determining deficits in activities of daily living and instrumental activities of daily living. Eight demonstrations made judgments regarding "risk of institutional placement," which also included assessment of clients' support systems and living arrangements. Four projects supplemented the functional assessment with indicators of cognitive impairment as targeting criteria. Four demonstrations (ACCESS, Georgia AHS, South Carolina, and New York Nursing Home Without Walls) required clients to be certified as eligible for skilled or intermediate level nursing home care. These are the same nursing home preadmission screening procedures required for nursing home admission within the respective states. This approach to targeting attempted to assure that project clients met all requirements for nursing home admission, even if they were never admitted. The Social/HMO, by contrast, is designed to enroll a representative population of frail, moderately impaired, and well elders. Here targeting is focused on enrolling specific percentages within each group in order to prevent adverse selection within a prepaid financing system. The demonstrations also targeted clients at two major transition points in the delivery system, discharge from hospitals and nursing homes.

Gatekeeping

Gatekeeping mechanisms are designed to control access to services, particularly high cost services. These mechanisms are used in developing and implementing care plans for clients. The most common gatekeeping approach in these demonstrations is the case managers' authority to prior authorize services covered by the waiver. The provision of waivered services for eligible clients could not be initiated without authorization from the project case manager. The most significant change in gatekeeping was the introduction of budget limitations and caps on the cost of individual client care plans, aggregate caseload costs, and/or aggregate agency costs. Eight demonstrations included budget caps as gatekeeping mechanisms, ranging from 75 percent to 85 percent of the costs of nursing home care. The presence of nursing home preadmission screening as a targeting method and the use of budget caps on care planning as a gatekeeping mechanism are features of both the more recent demonstrations and the Home and Community-Based Waiver Program in Medicaid.

Organizational Auspices

The organizational auspices for these demonstrations varied, with the largest number located in existing state agencies or existing provider agencies. Four projects operated from a newly created, independent, nonprofit agency base. One was hospital-based, two were in-home health agencies, and one project operated within a Health Maintenance Organization.

The preference for existing agencies and the limited use of newly created coordinating organizations reflects a number of design considerations. For example, in the early demonstration years (On Lok, Wisconsin CCO, Triage, ACCESS), project planners believed that it was necessary to create a new agency to administer newly available waivered services and to provide case management services. It was assumed that locating case management and direct service provision in the same organization would constitute a serious conflict of interest for the agency. These planners contended that case managers would be pressured, either directly or indirectly, to include their own agency's services in care plans and would have limited influence or control over the quality of service delivery. Later demonstration efforts were more commonly based in existing agencies, either government entities or community provider agencies.

AREA AGENCIES ON AGING

The Aging Network is the only national system of community-based agencies focused solely on the needs of elders. Area Agencies are responsible for planning, coordination, and delivery system development. As such, numerous Area Agencies have become involved with the delivery and/or funding of case management services. The National Association of Area Agencies on Aging (N4A) identified current innovative models of case management, which are presented in Table 8–2. These programs are illustrative of the types of initiatives undertaken by Area Agencies, but represent only a small portion of programs being implemented around the country.

Organizational Auspices

Four of the seven Area Agencies included in Table 8–2 are private, nonprofit organizations. Two are located in public agencies and one case management program (Dallas) is under contract with the Area Agency.

Targeting

Three of the case management programs require clients to be ICF or SNF certified. These programs also administer Medicaid Home) and Community-Based Waiver funds that require clients to be certified as meeting the nursing home level of care. The remainder of these programs use a variety of definitions of "frailty," "at risk," or "greatest need" as targeting criteria.

Gatekeeping and Financing

It is apparent from Table 8–2 that Area Agencies on Aging are less likely to function in a gatekeeping role. Further, where gatekeeping did occur, it was in the programs where the AAA was responsible for administering Medicaid funds. Projects with gatekeeping authority varied. Two had monthly budget caps for services. The Mid-Willamette AAA and the White River AAA had the ability to prior authorize waivered services. Mid-Willamette used preadmission

TABLE 8–2 Select Area Agency Case Management Experiences

Agency	Organizational Auspices	Target Population	Gatekeeping	Financing/ Reimbursement	Annual Budget (1984–85)
Mid-Willamette Senior Services Agency—Salem, Oregon	Private nonprofit AAA. Part of state-wide system which includes 2176 Waiver	Clients of "Closed Access Services" ICF/SNF certified	Preadmission screenings: prior authorization of waivered services	Medicaid/2176 Oregon Project Independence Older Americans Act	$1,489,410
Aroostook Area Agency on Aging, Presque Isle, Maine	Private nonprofit AAA. Part of state-wide system developed from state legislation & 2176 Waiver	Adults at risk of ICF, SNF or boarding home and seeking community placement	Monthly cap on individual budgets	Older Am. Act; Medicaid; State Administration funds; Social Services Block Grant; Maine Based Care Act; Private Fees; Local matching funds	$ 106,601
Region IV Area Agency on Aging—St. Joseph, Michigan	Private nonprofit AAA. State Unit on Aging funded demonstration project	Elderly at high risk of institutionalization	None	State Agency fund (ear-marked for case management demonstration); Older Am. Act Private Corporate Dollars	$ 118,000
ACCESS Center for the Elderly	Funded by Dallas AAA;	Older persons with difficult or	None	Older Americans Act; United	$ 130,721

Organization	Origin	Priority/Eligibility	Cost	Funding Source	Amount
(ACE)—Dallas, Texas	Outgrowth of Information and Referral project	multiple problems		Way; County Matching Funds	
Central Midlands Regional Planning Council—Columbia, South Carolina	Council of Governments sponsored AAA; developed as part of RWJ Foundation Health-Impaired Elderly Proj.	Priority to frail, homebound elderly	None	Robert Wood Johnson Foundation; Older Americans Act; Local and County matching funds	$ 151,650
Altamaha AAA—Baxley, Georgia	Area Planning and Development Commission sponsored AAA; part of statewide system developed from 1115 Waiver, st. legis., & 2176 Waiver	Functionally impaired adults; medicaid eligible; certified in need of nursing home care	$475 monthly cap	Medicaid & State Community Care Services Program; Older Americans Act	$ 69,000
White River AAA—Batesville, Arkansas	Private nonprofit AAA. Started as a State Long-Term Care Assessment and Referral demonstration project	Priority to elderly with greatest economic & social needs	Prior authorization for waivered services	State Service Management Funds	$ 192,819

screening to target resources to those most at risk of institutionalization.

The other three programs did not have gatekeeping as a case
management responsibility. They received their program funding
from the Older Americans Act; United Way; and private, foundation,
or other local government funds. The AAA experience here indicates
that gatekeeping at the AAA level, which is directly tied to the presence of Medicaid waivers, expands case managers' responsibilities.
Differences in the experiences of Area Agencies on Aging indicate
how the functions of case management are tied to the organizational
and financial structure of the program. In the absence of preadmission screening, cost caps, and/or capitated funding, gatekeeping is
not a case management function.

Another significant issue for Area Agency-based case management
programs is the question of whether case management is a "direct
service." In both the Dallas and Baxley, Georgia, agencies, case management was defined as a direct service. The Older Americans Act
prohibits Area Agencies from providing direct services. The Dallas
and Georgia agencies contracted for case management rather than
providing it through the area agency. The Dallas AAA contracted
with a provider agency and the Baxley, Georgia, agency developed
personal services contracts with individuals who served as case managers. In some states, case management has been defined as a direct
service and therefore outside the proper function of an area agency
on aging. In some states, like Connecticut, legislation mandates that
case management must be a separate service. In other states, case
management has not been defined as a direct service and Area Agencies on Aging directly provide the service. This determination varies
across the country, making it difficult to have a national case management system based in a single delivery system.

The ongoing work of local Area Agencies on Aging does not frequently receive attention. Innovative programming often goes unrec-
ognized, yet there is a rich experience that can be instructive to
program planners, administrators, and case managers. Each of the
Area Agency case management programs included in Table 8–2 is
described below. This previously unavailable information illustrates
the program variation that exists in a select group of area agencies on
aging.

Aroostook Area Agency on Aging; Presque Isle, Maine

The Aroostook AAA is the designated lead agency in its region for
implementation of Maine's "In-Home and Community Support Serv-

ices for Adults with Long-Term Care Needs Program," otherwise titled the Maine Home Based Care Program. The 1981 legislation called for competition for lead agency status. However, with the exception of one home health agency, all applicants were AAAs and in each area the AAA was, in fact, designated as the lead agency. Therefore, much of what is described for the Aroostook AAA could be generalized to the other Maine AAAs.

State legislation provided $1.25 million for the biennium (1984–1986) to increase the availability of in-home services. The Maine Department of Human Services also placed a moratorium on the construction of new nursing home beds. The Home Based Care legislation designated three priority groups: the elderly, physically handicapped nonelderly adults, and Adult Protective Services clients. The Department's Bureau of Maine's Elderly oversees approximately 75 percent of the total budget that was slated for the elderly.

Multidisciplinary teams were created and included at least one health and one social services professional to evaluate client needs and to develop and arrange plans of care. This "care management" was one component of the state legislation. Care management was defined as a planning, monitoring and advocating function designed to integrate and develop a comprehensive plan of in-home services based on the individual's needs. The plan is designed to maintain the older person's maximum independent functioning and to identify and resolve gaps in services (Aroostook, AAA, 1985). The Aroostook AAA also is the regional administrator of the Medicaid Alternative Long-Term Care Program. The policy of the AAA is to assure that Home Based Care funds are only used when Medicaid Waiver services cannot be utilized.

Within the Aroostook AAA structure, the multidisciplinary teams and assessment procedures vary according to whether the referral source is a hospital, home health agency, nursing home, boarding home, or other referral. After completing the assessment, the care manager develops a plan of care including cost estimates for one month's services. For Home-Based Care and Medicaid clients, the total care plan cannot exceed the state cap of the average cost of intermediate care facility services.

Formal reassessments are conducted every six months. Care managers review work orders and invoices submitted by service providers each month and compare them to the original authorizations before they approve payment. Care managers also have responsibility for brokering agreements and co-payment agreements, and serve as payroll agents between the client or family and contracted service provider. The client or family pays a 10 percent brokering agent fee to the Aroostook AAA. In the co-payment agreements, the clients or families are expected to contribute toward the cost of service as much as they are able. The AAA case manager monitors family compliance with what they had agreed to contribute. In the Payroll Agent agreements, the AAA acts as a payroll agent for clients or families who entered into the care management program and needed the services of a Personal Care Assistant. In all of the above situations, the care managers monitor payment, provision of services, contributions, and so forth. These various services are not limited to private pay clients. An income versus expenses assessment is completed and fees are assessed based on ability to pay. Stipends are available for low income persons.

The various components of case management are, in some instances, entirely the responsibility of the care manager. In other cases, personnel from other agencies are involved. The specific arrangement is dependent on the case and the referral source. A Quality Assurance Review Committee composed of hospital administrators, home care agencies, nursing home administrators, and others reviews policies for the program and periodically reviews randomly selected cases.

Care managers maintain average caseloads of 40 to 45 individuals. Case management costs were estimated to be $20.64 per hour. Care managers have to meet one of the following credential/experience requirements: certified by the state as an RN, hold a BA in social work with two years of experience, have a BA in human services with two years experience, or have eight years experience in direct service.

Central Midlands Regional Planning Council; Columbia, South Carolina

The Central Midlands AAA was one of eight grantees for the Robert Wood Johnson Foundation Program for the Health Impaired Elderly. All agencies under this program received five years of funding beginning in 1980. Each grantee was funded to develop a community-based central coordinating unit created by a formal joint agreement between the AAA and one or more voluntary agencies. The Central Midlands case management program was developed as part of the Health Impaired Elderly project.

The AAA defines this continuing case management program as to include the elements of comprehensive planning, coordinating, and monitoring of services. These are implemented to ensure that appropriate services are provided to meet the needs of the client (Central

Midlands Planning Council, 1984, p. 2). Needs assessment, eligibility determination, coordination and arranging of services, follow-up, and reassessment are identified as the major functions of the case management system.

The AAA maintains a central computerized client file system and provides technical assistance to community agencies. All other aspects of case management are contracted for with other agencies. A designated lead agency in each of the four counties is primarily responsible for case management. These lead agencies handle the majority of the cases. However, other agencies in this multiple entry system can also access the computerized system and provide ongoing case management. A central file of assessments is included in the Client Information data base.

The state of South Carolina's case management for its Title XIX waiver program is administered by the State Health and Human Services Department, separately from the AAA system. Case managers within the aging network arrange for a broad spectrum of community-based services funded by traditional sources. Persons eligible for Medicaid waivers are referred to the Health and Human Services program.

The average caseload size per case manager in the AAA system is unavailable, but the average cost of service is $16.41 per hour. In urban areas, a team is utilized for assessments; all other aspects of case management are carried out by case managers. In rural areas, case managers are solely responsible for all components. Staffing standards require a minimum of a BA to qualify as a case manager.

Dallas Area Agency on Aging; Dallas, Texas

Project ACE began in 1978 as an outgrowth of an information and referral service for senior citizens in Dallas. The Dallas AAA determined, through an analysis of service data, that persons most in need were not being served, because they were not being identified through existing outreach strategies. ACE is a network or consortium of 28 human service agencies in Dallas county that joined together to aid older persons with difficult or multiple problems. Five components are identified as key to the ACE program model: core staff, case management, ACE meetings, direct services network, and community resources.

The core staff includes a project director and three case managers. Case management involves a visit by the individual worker to the client's home to more adequately assess the overall situation including physiological, psychological, and environmental needs. After completing the assessment, a tentative case work plan is developed. The case manager then initiates and monitors the implementation of the plan (ACE Report, 1980). This agency identified four major case management functions: assessment, service plan development, linkage to services, and monitoring/follow-up.

Weekly ACE meetings were attended by core staff and representatives of the participating agencies. Meetings included discussion and assignment of proposed cases and preliminary case work plans. For some of the cases, a staff person from the other participating agencies served as the primary case manager and received assistance or backup from ACE core staff case managers. The referral source, including the AAA's Information and Referral program, carried out a preliminary assessment or screening. After discussion at the weekly meetings, final determinations of appropriateness for case management and specific assignment of responsibility were made.

The core staff case managers maintain average case loads of 135 individuals and broker the standard set of services available in the community. The program estimates case management costs at $9.20 per contact. Program staff were required to have a social services background, but specific skills were considered more critical than a specific educational degree.

After operating the ACE program for several years, the AAA decided to contract case management out to a community hospital social services department because of pressure from the State Unit on Aging (SUA), which viewed case management as an impermissible direct service. Under Older Americans Act regulations, AAAs are to provide direct services only under limited circumstances; however, the application of this regulation to case management varies from state to state. The Dallas AAA continues to maintain the project's information system, collecting the following data: client demographics (marital status, sex, race, age, income, zip code), problem categories, numbers of problems, referral sources, disposition, housing, and living arrangements.

Altamaha Area Agency on Aging; Baxley, Georgia

Georgia's current program of case management evolved from the Alternative Health Services Program, which was funded in 1976 as a 1115 Research and Demonstration waiver by the then Department of Health, Education and Welfare. Based on findings of that demonstration, the Georgia General Assembly included the program in the state's regular Medicaid program and allocated state matching funds. In 1981, the Georgia Department of Medical Assistance decided not to renew the 1115 Waiver, and instead applied for a Medicaid Waiver under the auspices of the Home- and Community-Based Waivers (2176) provision of the Omnibus Reconciliation Act of 1981. In 1982, the state legislature enacted Senate Bill 581, the "Community Care and Services for the Elderly Act." Among other things, this legislation transferred authority for case management and related services from the Medical Assistance department to the Office of Aging within the Georgia Department of Human Resources.

The Community Care Services Program has been available only to functionally impaired persons who are Medicaid eligible, or who will be eligible within 180 days of nursing home placement, who have health needs that can be adequately met in the community within established cost limits, and who desire to remain in the community. The cost cap is $475.00 per month.

State legislation requires that a minimum of six services be provided in each community care system. Four are mandated: assessment, case management, homemaker, and home health services. The other two could be any number of services, ranging from adult day care to senior center services to unspecified "other community services." In Georgia, case management is defined as "a management and administrative service which facilitates the process of planning, arranging, coordinating and evaluating service delivery to assure the most appropriate services are provided to the functionally impaired client in a timely and cost-effective manner" (Georgia Department of Human Resources, undated, p. I:11).

Teams consisting of a registered nurse and principal caseworker from District Public Health offices are responsible for initial screening and assessment. After an eligible person accepts the initial plan of care and enters the Community Care Services Program, he or she is referred to a case manager from the area's designated lead agency. The legislation creating the Community Care Program called for lead agencies in each of the state's 18 planning and service areas. Preference was given to AAAs in selecting lead agencies and, in fact, the AAA was designated the lead agency in each area. The lead agency either provides case management directly or subcontracts for its provision.

The Altamaha AAA services a 3,800 square mile region with over 21,000 older people in eight counties, and was one of the first Area Agencies in Georgia to provide case management. The AAA had planned to provide case management directly. A state Attorney General ruling, however, specified case management as a direct service, with planning and development commissions prohibited by state law from performing direct service. The AAA therefore opted to deliver case management through a personal services contract with an individual provider. Other AAAs in Georgia have similar arrangements.

The case manager has an active caseload of 132 clients. A second case manager has been added. Services obtained for clients are primarily Medicaid waivered services, but other community services are arranged as well. Case managers are required to have a BA in social services or certification as an RN, and have three years of relevant experience.

Mid-Willamette Valley Senior Services Agency;
Salem, Oregon

In Oregon, the designated State Unit on Aging (SUA) is the Senior Services Division (SSD), a section of the state Department of Human Resources. Oregon is currently the only state in the nation to have combined *all* state and federally funded programs for the elderly and long-term care into one state level agency and to create similar integration at the local level as well. The same state legislation created both the SSD at the state level and consolidated AAAs locally. Type A AAAs manage Older Americans Act and Oregon Project Independence funds only. Type B AAAs manage all the programs and funding sources available for older persons and persons under the age of 60 who are physically handicapped. Under a Type B arrangement, state eligibility workers and case workers transfer or work under contract to the AAA.

Oregon also heavily emphasizes deinstitutionalization and relocation with programs such as Nursing Home Relocation, Nursing Home Diversion, and Risk Intervention. Case management is described as a service designed to individualize and integrate social and health care options for *and* with the person being served. It attempts to assure appropriate levels of service and maximize coordination in the service delivery system. Four general components are included in their case management model; client entry, client assessment, service plan implementation and evaluation of client's response to services provided (Mid-Willamette AAA, 1985).

Entry into the Mid-Willamette case management system can come in the form of a written referral, letter, telephone call, or drop-in contact in any of four main offices or in one substation office. A service worker or service assistant conducts a preliminary screening to determine eligibility. Assessment is done in one of two ways. If the preliminary screening indicates that the client is at risk of nursing facility placement, a referral is made to the Pre-Admission Screening (PAS) team for assessment. The PAS team is composed of a Nurse,

Social Worker, and Service Worker. Exemptions from the required PAS assessment can be made for a Medicaid or Medicare eligible person who would require 21 days or less of nursing home care, and whose history confirms a substantive need for continuing nursing facility care, thereby ruling out the possibility of diversion. After the PAS team makes its recommendations for placement, the case file is forwarded to Mid-Willamette Service Workers for Service Plan finalization and implementation. If the preliminary screening does not indicate a risk of nursing facility placement, the assessment is conducted by a Service Worker, who also develops the service plan. At the assessment level, case management targeting criteria are not applied. However, prior to plan development and implementation, a person must have previously met eligibility criteria such as income, resources, and frailty.

All persons with potential for relocation are identified as such by marking their files, and these persons receive priority attention. There are two kinds of "flagging": Flagging/Relocation for cases where a client could be relocated to a lesser level of care within 30 days; and Flagging/Review, where more than 30 days would be required for relocation efforts to be completed. Case management clients living in their own homes or in adult foster homes are reassessed every six months. Case management clients living in nursing homes are reassessed once a year unless they have been "flagged."

Case managers with a nursing home case load average 180 to 200 clients; those with an in-home case load average 90 to 110 clients. Service costs are estimated to be $463.12 per client per month. Case managers primarily coordinate and arrange for services funded by the Medicaid waiver, Older Americans Act, and Oregon Project Independence. Workers must have a BA degree with two years experience in social services, or five years experience.

Region IV Area Agency on Aging, Inc.; St. Joseph, Michigan

In May of 1983, this AAA was the sole grant award recipient for the development and implementation of a case management service/research project from the Michigan Office of Services to the Aging. The AAA is a direct provider of case management under the grant. A research contract was negotiated with Western Michigan University to undertake the evaluation component.

Objectives of the Michigan project were: 1) to provide a single access point; 2) to assess emotional and health functioning; 3) to manage the coordination of existing services and programs; 4) to develop new services; and 5) to encourage and reward family support by arranging appropriate backup support from the traditional health and social services network.

Service functions within the program included: 1) serving a gatekeeper role within the continuum of care (within the context of this program, gatekeeper refers to access to service rather than setting caps or limits on service); 2) serving as a consultant to physicians; 3) brokering existing services; 4) providing client advocacy; 5) identifying unmet client needs; 6) coordinating formal and informal systems; 7) rewarding and encouraging informal support systems; 8) promoting community-based services; and 9) purchasing services on a one-time or short-term basis.

The program coordinator conducted initial eligibility screenings over the phone. The assessment and all other components of case management were done by a team consisting of a social worker and a nurse. The care plan required client and physician approval, and clients were reassessed at least every six months.

The initial team averaged 90 open cases during the first two years of operation. A second team was added in 1985. Qualification requirements for staff are an MSW or BSW for the social worker team member, and an RN for the nurse team member. Service costs were estimated at $643.00 per client per year. Services obtained for clients include the standard range of community services funded by Older Americans Act, Medicaid, United Way, etc., plus the direct purchase of some gap filling services with Older Americans Act and private corporate dollars.

White River Area Agency on Aging, Inc.; Batesville, Arkansas

The State of Arkansas has developed and issued case management guidelines for all Arkansas AAAs. The state defined case management as the "management of services through existing providers for those clients who need assistance with coordination of services in order for them to remain independent for as long as possible" (Arkansas Department of Human Services, 1984, p. 2). The target populations for case management were potential protective services clients (age 18 and over), and any older person (age 60 and over) who needed assistance through services existing within the community. Statewide implementation of case management through the area agency network began in 1983. Medicaid Personal Care program participants and current participants in AAA programs were considered initial priorities for case management services, the latter including home delivered meal participants. Prior to February 1984, target population priorities also included all participants at senior centers. The following basic case management elements were identified in the state guidelines: 1) written assessment; 2) care plan development; 3) documentation of implementation; and 4) periodic follow-up. The state provided considerable discretion to AAAs in implementing their case management programs.

Case management in the White River AAA began in 1982 as part of the Long-Term Care Assessment and Referral Project, which was authorized by the Arkansas legislature in 1981. White River was one of three sites for this demonstration that targeted Medicaid eligible clients. The project, with the overall goal of developing a comprehensive long-term care assessment system, included a Client Assessment Team. The team consisted of a consulting physician, an RN, a social worker, and a program director. Case managers were employed by the Client Assessment Team to channel each client through the assessment, referral, and service provision process.

White River AAA defines eleven units of service within its current case management program: assessment, counseling, evaluation, income support/material aid, information, interpreting-translation-letter writing, visiting, outreach, placement, referral, and telephoning.

The Information and Referral Specialists are responsible for prescreening, while all other components of case management are performed by case managers. Case loads average 180 per case manager. Case managers are required to have a BA in social services, or licensing by the state as a social worker. Three staff members are Licensed Practical Nurses. Clients receive services from the standard range of community services funded by the Older Americans Act, the United Way, and so on. Total program costs were estimated at $29.87 per client per hour.

MEDICAID HOME- AND COMMUNITY-BASED WAIVER PROGRAM (2176)

In 1981, Congress enacted Section 2176 of the Omnibus Budget Reconciliation Act (PL 97-35), which gave the Department of Health and Human Services the authority to grant to states a waiver of existing requirements of their Medicaid State Plans. Under this legislation, states could submit waiver applications that permitted the use of Medicaid funds for community-based long-term care services. Waivered Medicaid funds and services could only be provided to Medicaid eligible individuals who were assessed as nursing home certifiable at either the intermediate or skilled level of care. Section

2176 identified a package of services that states might offer in community-based long-term care plans: case management, home-maker services, home health aide services, personal care services, adult day health services, skilled nursing and rehabilitation, home-delivered meals, transportation, and respite care. Case management was defined in the regulations governing the 2176 waiver program as "a system under which responsibility for locating, coordinating, and monitoring a group of services rests with a designated person or organization" (Greenberg, Schmitz, & Lakin, 1983, p. 27).

The theory behind the 2176 waiver program is that home and community-based services can be substituted for more costly institutional services within the target groups served by the waiver and on an aggregate level.

> Perhaps the greatest significance of this program is that, for the first time, a range of health and personal care services and also case management are both specifically authorized in the legislation thus giving recognition to the social and medical aspects of long-term care under the Medicaid program (U.S. Senate Special Committee on Aging, 1982: p. 373).

Clients must be Medicaid eligible and must be determined to be "nursing home certifiable" by an objective assessment process. The assessment entails three separate determinations: level of care, appropriateness for home care, and care plan development to determine if the client can be maintained in the community for less than the individual care plan cost cap. The cost of the community care plan is controlled by placing a cap on allowable monthly expenditures, which is a specified percentage of the cost of institutional care that a person would receive if placed in a nursing home. For example, in the State of Washington, West Virginia, and Louisiana, the cap on community care plans is 80 percent of the cost of nursing home care. In Utah, New York, and Connecticut, the percentage is 75 percent, and in Kansas it is 90 percent.

Although most of the attention given to the 2176 waiver program has been focused on cost issues, it is clear that Congress also had other modifications in mind in the provision of long-term care services under the Medicaid program. The 2176 program is also intended to:

- establish nursing home preadmission screening programs to help prevent avoidable nursing home admissions;
- enhance continuity of care between institutional and community-based providers;

- require individualized care plans to enhance coordination;
- diversify services in order to enhance client choice;
- produce more thorough analyses of community care costs.

The use of Section 2176 waivers has become a key component of long-term care policy across the United States. One hundred and four 2176 waivers for aged/disabled programs (A/D) submitted by 41 states were approved by HCFA as of December 15, 1986. These waiver programs are diverse. Variations are evident in several key areas: services covered by the waiver, target populations, screening criteria, case management systems, service delivery networks, geographic areas covered, and reimbursement methods.

Case management is the most frequently provided service, with 85% of the 41 states with 2176 waiver programs including it in their service package, followed by homemaker services (65%), respite care (63%), adult day care (58%), and personal care (56%). In terms of breadth of services included in the waiver packages, 14 states provide five or fewer services, 21 states include between six and ten services, and 6 states deliver more than 10 services. Eligibility varies considerably across state 2176 waiver programs.

The 2176 program represents a major change in the way Medicaid funds can be expended, and incorporates case management functions as a major structural element in the waiver programs. The Home- and Community-Based Waiver program can be analyzed in terms of the four programmatic variables introduced earlier.

In terms of the four programmatic variables, the 2176 waiver programs can be summarized as indicated below:

Targeting: The target population for the Medicaid Home- and Community-Based Waiver program is Medicaid eligible clients (or those who would become eligible within a specified period) who, in the absence of services, would require the level of care provided in a skilled or intermediate care nursing home. The target population can also include current residents of nursing homes who could be safely deinstitutionalized and relocated to the community. Four client groups are identified: aged, disabled, mentally retarded, and mentally ill.

Gatekeeping: There are two major gatekeeping mechanisms in the 2176 program: nursing home preadmission screening (to determine the level of care), and the client care plan monthly budget caps. The monthly cap is a specified percentage of the monthly cost of nursing home care. In some states, there are also specific service utilization limitations. For example, in North Carolina, the cost of home mobility aides (grab bars, ramps) must not exceed $300 per year.

Funding/Reimbursement: For all of the 2176 programs, the source of funding is the Medicaid program, which is jointly financed by the federal and state governments. Medicaid is a welfare program designed to meet the health care needs of low income persons. Medicaid often becomes the payment source for older adults who enter nursing homes as private paying residents, liquidate their assets in order to cover the costs of their care, and spend down to the asset ceiling for Medicaid eligibility.

Organizational Auspices: The state Medicaid agency is responsible for administering the waiver program at the state level. Greenberg et al. (1983) reported, however, that in 45% of programs analyzed in 1983, three different organizations or levels of government were involved in determining client level of care, suitability for community care, and care plan development. Service delivery responsibility at the local level varies across the states with County Departments of Social Service or Health, or Area Agencies on Aging addressing the case management function. Contractual relationships with provider agencies are negotiated in order to arrange for the delivery of in-home and community-based services.

NEW INITIATIVES

Robert Wood Johnson Program in Hospital Initiatives in Long-Term Care

In 1982, the Robert Wood Johnson Foundation invested in a program of demonstration projects that was designed to stimulate hospitals to better provide for the health care needs of elders. The foundation recognized the significance of the relationship between the acute care, hospital discharge, and long-term care service delivery systems. Traditionally, the role of hospitals has been restricted to the period of time between the admission and discharge; however, with the advent of DRGs, length of stay and timeliness of discharge have become critical elements in hospitals' financial status. Shorter lengths of stay and lower occupancy rates have motivated many hospitals to expand their service repertoire to include continuing and long-term care. Vertical integration has become a rather widespread response from hospitals whose acute care product line alone does not bring in sufficient revenue.

The Robert Wood Johnson Hospital Initiatives in Long-Term Care Program anticipated and sought to stimulate such developments. Twenty-four sites have been in operation since 1983. The hospitals awarded grants are a very diverse group, including both public and

TABLE 8–3 Location of Project Sites

• Craven County Hospital Corporation New Bern, North Carolina	• Cuyahoga County Medical System Cleveland, Ohio
• San Francisco Dept. Public Health San Francisco, California	• South Shore Hospital Miami, Florida
• Good Samaritan Hospital Puyallup, Washington	• Intermountain Health Care, Inc. Richfield, Utah
• Johns Hopkins Hospital Baltimore, Maryland	• Kuakini Medical Center Honolulu, Hawaii
• Massachusetts General Hospital Boston, Massachusetts	• Meharry Medical College Nashville, Tennessee
• Morristown Memorial Hospital Morristown, New Jersey	• Mount Sinai Hospital Hartford, Connecticut
• Mount Sinai Medical Center Milwaukee, Wisconsin	• Mount Zion Hospital San Francisco, California
• Parkland Memorial Hospital Dallas, Texas	• Senior Health Plan, Inc. St. Paul, Minnesota
• St. Luke's Medical Center Boise, Idaho	• St. Vincent's Medical Center New York, New York
• UCLA Medical Center Los Angeles, California	• University Hospital Boston, Massachusetts
• University of Maryland Medical System Baltimore, Maryland	• University of Virginia Hospitals Charlottesville, Virginia
• Valley Lutheran Hospital Mesa, Arizona	• West Virginia University Morgantown, West Virginia

Funding for these projects terminated at the end of 1987. An evaluation contract was awarded to the Bigel Institute at Brandeis University. The evaluation study focuses on several substantive areas including: case mix and client level; case management; financial viability; and organizational, professional, and workplace impacts.

private, small community hospitals, and tertiary care university-based teaching hospitals in rural, urban, and suburban locations (see Table 8–3). Evaluation of findings highlight the diversity of case management practice in the various hospital sites. Four program models were identified: nursing home diversion, aftercare management, medical management, and community care coordination (Capitman, et.al., 1988). Variations in organizational features and client care mix were also noted as significant program dimensions.

LONG-TERM CARE INSURANCE

As pressures on public funding for long-term care services mount, there has been growing interest in developing private long-term care insurance. While there is some disagreement regarding the capacity of private long-term care insurance to provide significant protection for elders (Wiener, Rivlin, Hanley, Spence, 1988), increasing interest in this area continues to expand the array of insurance products available. At present, insurance options include three major types: individually-marketed indemnity policies, continuing care retirement communities, and consolidated delivery systems such as the model used in the Social/HMO.

Most insurance coverage provides benefits limited to extended nursing home (skilled and intermediate) care stays and is based on indemnity policies that pay a fixed amount per day for covered services. Most policies also include a deductible or a reduced benefit over time. Premiums are age-rated and policies often require a three-day hospitalization prior to admission to a nursing home.

The inclusion of home health benefits in long-term care insurance policies is a relatively new development. Insurers have been reluctant to cover home health care because they fear insurance-induced demand. In the absence of a home health benefit, however, long-term care insurance policies will create an incentive for institutional placement. Further, since nursing home placement is a distasteful option for most elders, including home health benefits can be useful as a marketing strategy. In the absence of a strong case management mechanism, insurers are reluctant to liberalize coverage and include home health benefits.

A major deviation from the traditional indemnity approach involves combining insurance and service delivery (Social/HMO, Continuing Care Retirement Communities, Metropolitan Life/Group Health Cooperative of Puget Sound). In these situations, the provider is also the insurer, an arrangement that provides an incentive to keep service delivery in line with available resources. By delivering care more efficiently, these insurance and service delivery combinations seek to reduce the financial risks of insuring long-term care. Where providers are at risk, case management can be used as a primary risk management strategy.

These managed-care systems employ case managers to screen, certify, assess, and develop care plans in collaboration with clients. Care plans are developed within strict cost limits and are closely scrutinized by supervisors. Incentives in the care planning process are designed to keep clients in their homes through the provision of home and community-based services. Case managers have the authority to directly order, monitor, and terminate services on behalf of their clients. The presence of provider risk creates pressures to increase the reliability and predictability of case management practice. Leutz et al. (1985) specified a number of areas in which case management practice will be standardized in the Social/HMO sites: standardizing assessment instruments and processes; defining service objectives in care plans; developing criteria for care plan decisions; recruitment, socialization, training, and supervision; and classifying clients.

CASE MANAGEMENT MODELS

Past, present, and future approaches to financing and delivering long-term care services have included and will continue to include some form of case management. The operational experiences described in this chapter demonstrate the evolution of case management across time, organizational types, and financing strategies (see Table 8–4).

These case management models are shaped by the nature of program financing. As case managers are given greater authority for developing fiscally responsible care plans, the nature of the job will become increasingly complex, requiring higher levels of accountability. It is reasonable to expect that the greater the provider risk, the tighter the control over care planning and other program costs.

Program development, implementation, and evaluation efforts must be model specific. Only in this way is it possible to compare the relative effectiveness of the different case management models. Prior to considering program outcomes, however, it is necessary to have

TABLE 8–4 Model Characteristics

Broker	Service Management	Managed Care
	model 1:	
• no service $	• preadmission screening	• prospective funding
• no budget caps	• authorize waivered services	• provider risk
• referrals	• budget caps	• preadmission screening
• follow-up		• budget caps
• adovocacy with providers		
	model 2:	
	• no preadmission screening	
	• budget caps	
	• authorize waivered services	

thorough knowledge of program inputs. Just what kind of case management is provided? The answer to this question, perhaps based on the models described in this volume, represents a critical step in the design, implementation, and evaluation phases of a comprehensive program planning process.

Chapter **9**

Issues in Planning a Case Management Program

Throughout this volume a series of issues critical to designing and evaluating long-term care case management programs has been presented. The experiences of the long-term care demonstrations and ongoing programs reviewed indicate that a range of program options exist in developing and implementing case-managed care, and that the success of the case management intervention is dependent on a thorough analysis of these program options. To this end, this final chapter summarizes responses to several key questions that should be addressed when planning a system of case-managed care. These diagnostic questions, which need to be considered by organizations or systems exploring the use of case management, fall into the following major categories:

- Definition and Rationale for Long-Term Care Case Management
- Environmental Context of Case Management
- The Role of Case Management: Reflection of Program Goals
- Technology of Case Management
- Costs of Case Management
- Quality Assurance and Evaluation of Case Management.

DEFINITION AND RATIONALE FOR LONG-TERM CARE CASE MANAGEMENT

Two initial questions must be addressed by organizations or delivery systems considering the development of a case-managed program: (1) How will long-term care case management be defined? and (2) What is the rationale for installing case management within an agency or delivery system? These questions are critical because there has been both considerable confusion in defining case management and a lack of clarity in expectations concerning the effects of case-managed care.

As noted in Chapter 1, long-term care case management is an intense, comprehensive, and long-term intervention directed at a chronically impaired population of individuals. This definition implies that the case management intervention requires relatively small case-loads, a comprehensive approach to assessment and care planning, and an ongoing monitoring component not tied to the provision of a specific service. Although a number of service providers manage the services that they provide to their clients, this approach is distinct from long-term care case management, which has greater breadth of coverage, encompassing the range of community-based services needed by impaired individuals. Thus, clearly defining the type of case management intervention to be implemented is a key step. Case management as defined above is only one potential option for coordinating, delivering, and controlling access to services. There are other forms of case management, such as those programs that arrange an initial package of services and then allow the client and family to manage their own care from that point. Some programs have trained family members to perform the case management role while others have varied the intensity of the case management depending on the client's level of disability and family supports available.

In addition to case management, there are numerous other approaches to distributing and managing a long-term care benefit, such as expansion of the current Medicare coverage, the use of vouchers for services, or even direct cash payments to clients and families to purchase services on their own. The decision on how to coordinate and manage the long-term care services in a community must be considered carefully.

Understanding the nature and definitions of the case management intervention is not enough. Recognizing what case management can and cannot accomplish is also essential. Some proponents of case management believe that it has been a solution to all of the ills of the long-term care system. Indeed, case management is a technique to aid in gaining access to, coordinating, and monitoring the system of care; however, it cannot cure the problems caused by the lack of a comprehensive long-term care policy or the lack of long-term care financing. Case management can be part of a system reform process, but without linking case management to other system components such as preadmission screening, long-term care bed supply, and financing, case management will have a limited effect on the service delivery system.

ENVIRONMENTAL CONTEXT OF CASE MANAGEMENT

As suggested above, it is critical to recognize that any case management intervention will be imbedded in a complex environment that includes a myriad of federal, state, and local policies; a variety of providers; and a range of resources. For example, case management will not be a terribly effective intervention in an environment in which there is an extreme shortage of services. However, developing

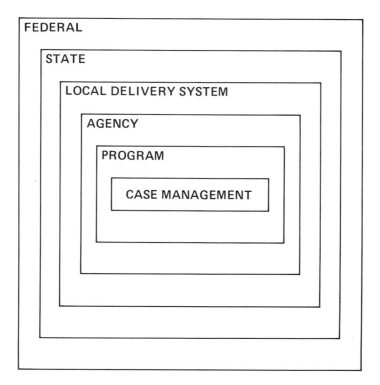

Figure 9–1 Environmental context of case management.

a case management system may make considerable sense in an environment in which a range of services exists without the benefit of a coordinating agency.

Figure 9–1 provides a model for examining case management in the context of the environment. Case management, in the center of the model, is affected by each of the outlying concentric boxes. For example, state funding for long-term care services, the nature of the local delivery system, and local agency operations all represent important factors that will shape the case management system to be implemented. This highlights the importance of examining case management in the context of the existing system. Again, it must be emphasized that case management does not exist in a vacuum, but rather in the center of a complex system of care that may include conflicting elements and pressures. Decisions concerning the role, technology, and financing of case management are particularly dependent on these outer dimensions.

THE ROLE OF CASE MANAGEMENT: REFLECTION OF PROGRAM GOALS

The roles and responsibilities of case management can vary considerably depending on program or system objectives. For instance: Is the case management system designed to control access to the community-based long-term care system? Is the case management system designed to authorize or control expenditures on community-based services? Is the case management system designed to control access or benefits to institutional care? Is the case management system designed to advocate for the needs of chronically impaired individuals? Is case management a mandatory or voluntary intervention? Who is the case manager supposed to serve?

It is clear that case management has developed multiple roles with an emphasis on advocacy and coordination, expansion of care benefits, and gatekeeping and benefit control. These roles, which may present conflicts for individual case managers or an entire organization, must be considered carefully in the design of a program. For example, the potential for conflict between the advocacy and gatekeeping roles is particularly strong, and yet this dual role has become a major element of case management practice in many of the programs reviewed. As noted earlier, both the service management and managed-care models use case managers to advocate for client needs and control the amount of dollars expended on services. It is reasonable to ask case managers to perform multiple roles; however, it is also essential to provide adequate training and support in the performance of these activities. Without proper training and support, the multiple responsibilities faced by case managers can become considerably destructive to program operations.

As discussed throughout this book, the level of case manager authority is a key program component. The three models examined represent very different roles and responsibilities for the case managers and the organization. The scope of case manager authority can vary widely, ranging from the use of volunteer nonprofessional case managers with no control over resources to highly trained professionals with the organizational ability to assemble packages of acute care as well as community and institutional long-term care benefits. This authority also pertains to monitoring these services as well as terminating client benefits. Matching case manager responsibilities to program objectives is thus critical in the design of a case management intervention. A poor match between case manager roles and program objectives will ensure dissatisfaction with the case management intervention.

TECHNOLOGY OF CASE MANAGEMENT

Designing a case management program involves a series of strategic decisions about the core case management intervention. Issues that must be addressed include: structure of the core functions, staffing and supervisory patterns, training and professional orientation for case managers, location of the case management organization, establishment of standards of care, interface with acute-health-care providers, and involvement of caregivers and clients as consumers.

Decisions regarding the technology of case management are directly linked to the type of model of case-managed care implemented. For example, if case management is to serve as a preadmission screening unit, the assessment process has to be designed both to determine eligibility and to provide information so that a comprehensive care plan can be developed. Such a responsibility also has implications for staffing, training, supervision, agency structure, information system structure, and quality assurance and evaluative responsibilities. Similarly, if a case management program is serving a slightly less disabled population, the assessment process may be somewhat different. The key point is that case management technology needs to be continually tied to the agency's objectives, environment, and roles of the case management intervention.

There are a number of questions that consistently arise surrounding the technology of case management. From the selection of assessment instrumentation, to staffing, to monitoring mechanisms, case management agencies face a series of decisions concerning program implementation. Some of the most common technological issues in case management are reviewed in this section.

Targeting Case Management to the Right People

Targeting case-managed community care to the right population has been a major issue in long-term care ever since the first community care demonstration was initiated in 1973. The long-term care demonstrations consistently reported difficulties in targeting clients who were at risk of nursing home placement and many cited this as a weakness of these projects (Weissert, 1985b). It is true that the vast majority of demonstrations had difficulties identifying individuals who would have entered a nursing home without the benefit of case-managed care. However, a review of these studies indicates that over time the projects were indeed able to serve a more impaired clientele in need of long-term care. The demonstration projects and ongoing programs have improved in their ability to serve more disabled clients, and in that regard their targeting efforts have improved. Identifying which highly disabled persons will reside in institutional settings and which persons will remain in the community remains a difficult challenge. But it is not clear that this represents a targeting failure. For every nursing home resident there are approximately two people in the community with comparable levels of impairment (Kunkel & Applebaum, 1990). Perhaps the long-term care system should be designed to meet the needs of all those individuals with chronic disabilities without regard to their choice of setting for the care they need.

If a program adopts a philosophy of serving those with long-term needs without regard to whether nursing home placement is imminent, then targeting based on functional disability is recommended. Although it is important to consider other aspects of clients' lives, such as living arrangements, availability of informal supports, environment, and attitudes toward care, functional ability should be the main criterion for targeting case-managed care. Using functional eligibility criteria is a mechanism with proven effectiveness in ensuring that a needy population is being served by the case management program.

Client Assessment

One of the most common questions raised by organizations involves client assessment. Both the research and practice communities have spent a considerable amount of time searching for the optimum assessment process. Although the assessment process is important and a poor tool can clearly have a negative influence on practice, it is our contention that assessment has received too much emphasis relative to the other case management functions. For example, despite our emphasis on assessment, we have spent very little time improving the process of translating this information into a comprehensive plan of care. At this point, there are numerous assessment tools already developed and we recommend adopting or adapting existing instrumentation rather than spending resources developing a completely new instrument.

Professional Orientation and Training for Case Managers

Another issue that typically arises involves professional orientation, education, and training of case managers. The opinion on professional orientation is split, with some arguing that nurses should be case managers and others feeling equally strongly that social workers should be used for the job. Because long-term care represents an interface between health and social services, both nurses and social workers can perform the case management tasks well. It is clear that each of these two professions can benefit by working together to draw upon the expertise of other related disciplines. For example, social work case managers must have adequate health training to properly serve highly disabled people who commonly experience significant health problems. Similarly, there are important aspects of social work training, such as understanding the structure and availability of the service system and understanding the intricacies of family relations, that are essential to good case management practice. Thus, while there is no one profession best suited to perform case management tasks, case managers do need to have training in several important areas.

Based on the experience of previous long-term care demonstrations, three areas of training have been identified as important for case managers (Applebaum & Wilson, 1988). The first training category involves the need to understand clients and includes knowledge of health and disability limitations, morbidity and mortality patterns, and mental health needs. Even though many case managers have had some previous training and experience, the frailty of those receiving long-term care poses some unanticipated challenges. High rates of morbidity and mortality mean that case managers require considerable knowledge about health conditions. Additionally, many case managers need substantial emotional support because of the high mortality rates that are common in this population.

A second category of training needs is associated with understanding the service environment. This category comprises awareness of service providers, eligibility criteria, and service unit costs; methods of negotiating with and monitoring providers working with physicians and other medical personnel; and knowledge of support mechanisms for informal caregivers. The third category encompasses techniques of case management including the core case management functions of assessment, care planning, and ongoing monitoring as well as methods for balancing the multiple case manager roles and time management. Our experience suggests that, in addition to the standard professional training received by social workers, nurses, and other human service professionals, case managers require a special combination of skills and experiences.

How Case Management Should Be Organized

A major issue surrounding the provision of case management is what type of agency should provide case-managed care. Since the development of the concept of case management, there has been an ongoing debate about whether case managers should be located in free-standing organizations not responsible for the provision of specific services, or as part of a service-providing organization. Some have argued that the strength of case management lies in its independent operation and the freedom it affords case managers to choose the optimum service packages without constraints. For example, several states, such as Connecticut, have legislatively mandated that case management must be provided by an agency not responsible for providing direct home care services such as home health aide, nursing, meals, or transportation. An alternative perspective is that since certain service providers, such as home health agencies, spend considerable time in clients' homes, they are in a much better position to manage the care provided. Whether the agency is a direct-service provider can be an important factor, but this should not be the sole determinant of location. In fact, other criteria, such as agency reputation in the community, past experience with the long-term care population, the quality of services provided, and management ability appear to be of greater importance. The key point, however, is that the case management unit must be able to choose services and providers independently. Prohibiting the integration of case management and direct service providers is one method to ensure this independence, but not the only method. However the separation between case management and service provision is achieved, case managers must be able to be independent in arranging and monitoring a plan of care.

Client Family Involvement with the Case Manager

Because a large proportion of community-based long-term care is provided by family members, case managers' interactions with the informal system are critical to good practice. The challenge is to support rather than supplant the informal system while providing care to disabled relatives and friends. Case managers, particularly in models that include control over a substantial amount of community resources, can have an important effect on family roles and responsibilities. Case managers have to be cognizant of the effects of new services on clients and their families. For example, arranging a home-delivered meal for the husband being cared for by his frail wife may seem like a good service. However, if preparing her husband's meal was one of the wife's major caregiving tasks, this could have a negative effect on the couple. Similarly, bringing in a formal service that had traditionally been completed by a visiting family member may reduce some important family interaction.

Balancing the services to be provided by the informal and formal systems is indeed a significant challenge faced in case management. Research evidence from the National Channeling Demonstration has provided some positive evidence concerning this interface. One of the research components of the demonstration evaluated the effects on the informal care system of expanding case-managed services. One major finding of that study was that there was very little substitution of formal for informal care despite increases in the amount of dollars spent on services. This finding has been reinforced in several other studies as well (Christianson, 1986). This evidence suggests that families continue to assume major responsibility for community long-term care. Therefore, case managers must carefully observe how their intervention affects family roles and responsibilities.

COSTS OF CASE MANAGEMENT

There is considerable interest in the costs associated with the case management intervention. The definition of case management has varied considerably, and thus so have estimates of its cost. It is clear that a case management program with a caseload of 300 clients per case manager will have substantially different costs than a program in which a case manager is responsible for only 50 clients. Case management intervention costs are also affected by a series of other factors, such as the type of clientele served (level of disability), responsibilities of the case managers (for example, whether or not they perform a nursing home preadmission screen), the geographic area served by the program, organizational structure, and type of personnel used.

Information on the costs of case management in ongoing programs has not generally been reported; however, several of the long-term care demonstrations have reported such cost information. An examination of the cost results from six long-term care demonstrations (Haskins et al 1985; Thornton et al., 1986) reported that the monthly costs for case management ranged from $49 to $145 per client each month. Members of the BPA study team responsible for evaluating five of the demonstrations suggested that the largest variation in the costs of case management was due to differences in the amount of staff time spent with each client. For example, the South Carolina Long-Term Care Project emphasized nursing home preadmission screening of applicants much more extensively than ongoing case management. After enrollment, case managers had less contact with clients than in some of the other projects, due to their larger caseloads. BPA suggested that cost differences also resulted from variations in the level of staff professionalization, degree of specialization, differences in local environments, size of the catchment area, and the number and type of local providers.

Results from the 10 sites of the National Channeling Demonstration showed case management costs ranging from $88 to $120 per month with an average of $102 per client month. Channeling researchers divided costs between the initial functions of screening, assessment, care planning, and ongoing case management. The cost of the initial functions (screening, assessment, care planning) averaged $206 per month. When combined with the costs of administrative and clerical tasks, the total cost associated with the initial case management functions including agency overhead was $340 per client. The ongoing costs of case management, which included those activities conducted after the completion of the initial functions, averaged $89 per month. When combined with the initial functions, this resulted in an average cost per client of $102 per month.

Costs of ongoing programs may vary from the costs of these demonstration projects; however, these numbers do indicate that long-term care case management is an intensive effort with specific costs associated with the intervention. Although case management costs in these projects represented a relatively small proportion of the total service dollars spent (10–20%), these costs suggest that a case management intervention will require significant resources. Whether the resources that have been invested in case management will help manage the community-based care benefit is thus the crucial cost-benefit question to be addressed. Unfortunately, this question has not been researched thus far.

A second issue that arises when discussing the costs of case management is that of whether case management is a service or an administrative function. Some programs (Austin et al., 1985) have viewed case management as a separate community-based service, comparable in nature to other in-home services such as home health aide, nursing, and home delivered meals. Other programs have considered case management an administrative mechanism that manages the direct provision of community-based services. Although classifying case management as either an administrative effort or a service program has important implications for reimbursement, it seems to have a very small effect on program structure or effectiveness. It appears that programs or systems have defined case management based on reimbursement maximization rather than on program philosophy. Our review suggests that as long as the key principles of case management are established, whether these activities are considered as an administrative practice or as a separate service is not particularly important.

QUALITY ASSURANCE AND EVALUATION OF CASE MANAGEMENT

A critical question faced in developing a case management program is, how do you ensure the quality of case-managed care? This task is difficult because case management includes two distinct but related components: the core case management activities and also the specific services monitored but not provided by the case management agency. In order for case management to be a successful intervention, both the case management activities and the direct services must be provided effectively. Thus, evaluative and quality assurance activities should address both components of managed care.

Throughout the second part of this book evaluative activities have been divided into two categories: evaluation and quality assurance. A case management intervention should include both evaluation and quality assurance activities into its operational activities. Figure 9–2 provides an example of the quality assurance and evaluation interface. Quality in this figure is viewed as the product of impact evaluation (knowing that the intervention works) and quality assurance (ensuring that the program is implemented according to standards).

Case management programs should have a strategic plan in which evaluation and quality assurance activities are integrated. The case management intervention must be subjected to impact evaluation to establish the validity of the intervention. However, after validity of the intervention has been established, a quality assurance system

Quality Circle

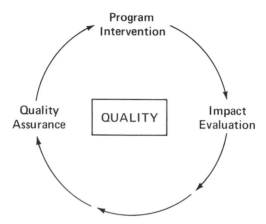

Figure 9–2 Integrating quality assurance.

should also become part of ongoing practice. This quality assurance effort must focus both on case management activities and the direct services coordinated by the case managers.

With growing pressure in the future to serve clients with higher and higher levels of disability as cost consciously as possible, quality assurance will likely be the major issue facing case management agencies for years to come.

References

Abrahams, R., & Leutz, W. (1983). The consolidated model of case management and service provision to the elderly. *Pride Institute Journal of Long-Term Home Health Care*, 2(4), 29–34.

Access Center for the Elderly, ACE (1980). "Annual Report" Dallas, TX: Community Council of Greater Dallas/Dallas Area Agency on Aging.

Amerman, E. (1983). The nurse/social worker dyad in community-based long-term care. Presented at the Annual Meeting of the Gerontological Society of America, Nov., San Francisco, CA. For a description of how the Philadelphia Channeling Project designed its program to address this potential problem.

Amerman, E., Eisenberg, E., & Weisman, R. (1983). Case management and counseling: A service dilemma experience from channeling. Paper presented at the 36th Annual Meeting of The Gerontological Society of America, San Francisco.

Applebaum, R. (1989). What's all this about quality? *Generations XIII* (1):5–7.

Applebaum, R. (1988). Recruitment and Characteristics of Channeling Clients, *Health Services Research*, Vol 23, Number 1 (April) pg 51–66.

Applebaum, R., Atchley, S., McGinnis, R., Bare, A. (1988). *A guide to ensuring the quality of in-home care.* Columbus, OH: Ohio Department of Aging.

Applebaum, R., Austin, C.D., & Atchley, R. (1987). *Ohio's passport program: A program review.* Scripps Gerontology Center, Miami University and College of Social Work, Ohio State University, Columbus, Ohio.

Applebaum, R., & Harrigan, M. (1986). *Channeling effects on the quality of clients' lives.* Princeton, NJ: Mathematica Policy Research.

Applebaum, R., Harrigan, M., & Kemper, P. (May 1986). The evaluation of the national long-term care demonstration: Tables comparing channeling to other community care demonstrations. Princeton, NJ: Mathematica Policy Research.

Applebaum, R., & Wilson, N. (1988). Training needs for providing case management for the long-term care client: Lessons from the National Channeling Demonstration. *The Gerontologist, 28*(2):172–176.

Arkansas Department of Human Services, Office on Aging (1984). Comprehensive case management guidelines. Little Rock, AR.

Aroostook Area Agency on Aging, Inc. (1985). 1985 Amended Maine Home Based Care Regional Plan. Presque Isle, ME.

Austin, C.D. (1983). Case management in long-term care: Option and opportunities. *Health and Social Work, 8*(1):16–30.

Austin, C.D. (1984). Penny wise and pound foolish: What is the future of long-term care? Presented at International Institute of Sociology, 13th World Congress, Sept., Seattle, WA.

Austin, C.D., Roberts, L., & Low, J. (1985). *Case management: A critical review.* Seattle, WA: University of Washington, Institute on Aging.

Baxter, R.J., Applebaum, R., Callahan, Jr., J.J., Christianson, J.B., & Day, S.L. (April 15, 1983). *The planning and implementation of channeling: Early experiences of the National Long-Term Care demonstration.* Washington, DC: Mathematica Policy Research.

Beatrice, D.F. (1981). Case management: A policy option for long-term care. In Callahan and Wallack (eds), *Reforming the long-term care system.* Lexington, MA: D.C. Heath, Lexington Books.

Birnbaum, H., Gaumer, G., Pratter, F., & Burke, R. (Dec. 1985). Nursing home without walls: Evaluation of the New York State Long-Term Home Health Program. Contract No. 500-79-0052. Prepared for Health Care Financing Administration. Cambridge, Mass. Abt Associates.

Branch, L., & Jette, A. (1982). A prospective study of long-term care institutionalization among the aged. *American Journal of Public Health, 72*(12): 1373–1379.

Brown, R., Schore, J,. Wooldridge, J., & Madison, W. (1984). Hospital and nursing home use and mortality. Presented at 37th Annual Meeting of the Gerontological Society of America, Nov., San Antonio, TX.

Burack-Weiss, A. (1988). Clinical aspects of case management. *Generations XII*(5): 23–25.

Callahan, J.J., & Wallack, S.S. (1981). *Reforming the Long-Term-Care System.* Lexington, MA: Lexington Books.

Capitman, J.B., MacAden, M., & Yee, D. (1988). Hospital-based case management. *Generations XII*(5): 62–65.

Capitman, J.B., Haskins, B., & DeGraaf, B. (June 1983). *Preliminary report on work in progress: Evaluation of coordinated community-oriented long-term care demonstration projects.* Berkeley, CA: Berkeley Planning Associates.

Carcagno, G.J., Applebaum, R., Christianson, J., Phillips, B., & Thornton, C. (July 1986). The evaluation of the National Long-Term Care Demonstration: The planning and operational experience of the Channeling projects. Princeton, NJ: Mathematica Policy Research.

Christianson, J.B. (1988) The Evaluation of National Long-Term Care Demonstration: The Effect of Channeling on Informal Caregivers, Health Services Research, Vol 23, Number 1, pgs. 99–199.

Coale, C. (1983). Care for the elderly: Fiscal accountability in a case managed system. Paper presented at the Gerontological Society of America, San Francisco.

Crosby, P.B. (1979). *Quality is free: The art of making quality certain.* New York: McGraw-Hill.

Donabedian, A. (1966). Evaluating the quality of medical care. *Milbank Memorial Fund Quarterly* 44(3): 166–206.

Dronska, H. (1983). Focus: The role of case management in long-term home health care. *Pride Institute Journal of Long-Term Home Health Care*, 2(4): 21–28.

Eggert, G.M., et al. (1986). *Direct assessment vs. brokerage: A comparison of case management models.* Monroe County Long-Term Care Program/Access.

George, L.K., & Landerman, R. (1982). *Health and life satisfaction: A replicated secondary data analysis.* Durham, NC: Duke University Center for the Study of Aging and Human Development.

Georgia Department of Human Resources (no date). *Case management and community care for the elderly (training manual).* Atlanta, GA.

Gottesman, L.E., Ishizaki, B., & MacBride, S.M. (1979). Service management: Plan and concept in Pennsylvania. *The Gerontologist,* 19(4): 379–385.

Greenberg, J.N., Doth, D.S., & Austin, C.D. (Nov. 1981). A comparative study of long-term care demonstrations: Lessons for future inquiry. University of Minnesota: Center for Health Service Research.

Greenberg, J.N., Schmitz, M.P., & Lakin, C.K. (June 1983). *An analysis of responses to the medicaid Home- and Community-Based Long-Term Care Waiver Program (section 2176 of P1 97-35).* Washington, D.C.: National Governors' Association, State Medicaid Information Center.

Grinnell, R.M. (1981). *Social work research and evaluation.* Itasca, IL: F.E. Peacock Publishers, Inc.

Grisham, M. (1983). Case management for the frail elderly: Expected caseload size for a caseload of clients on the threshold of institutionalization. Presented at the 111th Annual Meeting of APHA, Nov. 13–17, Dallas, TX.

Grisham, M., & White, M. (1982). Issues in interdisciplinary case management: Composition, supervision, workload. Presented at the 110th Annual Meeting of APHA, Nov. 14–18, Montreal, Quebec, Canada.

Haskins, B., Capitman, J.B., Collignon, F., DeGraaf, B., & Yordi, C. (1985). Evaluation of coordinated community oriented long-term care demonstrations. Contract No. 500-80-0073. Prepared for Health Care Financing Administration. Berkeley, CA: Berkeley Planning Associates.

Health Impaired Elderly Project (1984). *Case management for the elderly: A manual of procedures.* Columbia, S.C.: Central Midlands Regional Planning Council.

Institute on Aging (1987). Improving Access for Elders: The Role of Case Management Final Report. University of Washington, Seattle, Washington.

Interstudy (1986). *A description and analysis of state pre-admission screening programs*. Excelsior, MN.

Johnson, M.L., & Sterthous, L.M. (1982). *A guide to memorandum of understanding negotiation and development for long-term care management agencies*. Philadelphia, PA: Mid-Atlantic Long-Term Care Gerontology Center, Temple University.

Kane, R.A., & Kane, R.L. (1981). *Assessing the elderly: A practical guide*. Lexington, MA: Lexington Books.

Kane, R.A., & Kane, R.L. (1987). *Long-term care: Principles, programs and policies*. New York: Springer.

Kemper, P., Applebaum, R., & Harrigan, M. (1987). A systematic comparison of community care demonstrations. Madison, Wisconsin: University of Wisconsin Institute for Research on Poverty.

Kemper, P., Applebaum, R., Brown, R.S., Carcagno, C.G., Christianson, J., Grannemann, T., Harrigan, M., Holden, N., Phillips, B., Schore, J., Thornton, C., & Woodbridge, J. (1986). *The evaluation of the National Long-Term Care Demonstration. Final Report*. Princeton: Mathematica Policy Research.

Kunkel, S., & Applebaum, R. (1990) Estimating the Prevalence of Long-Term Disability for an Aging Society, unpublished.

Kodner, D.L., Mossey, W., & Dapello, R.D. (1984). New York's "Nursing Home Without Walls": A provider-based community care program for the elderly. In R.T. Zawadski (ed.), *Community-based systems of long-term care*. New York: The Haworth Press.

Leutz, W., Greenberg, J.N., Abrahams, R., Prottes, J., Diamond, L., & Gruenberg, L. (1985). *Changing health care for an aging society: planning for the social HMO*. Boston, MA: Lexington Press.

Mid-Willamette Valley Senior Services Agency (1985), (Internal Document). Salem, OR.

Miller, L., Clark, M., & Walter, L., (1984). The comparative evaluation of the Multipurpose Senior Services Project—1981–1982: Final Report. Grant No. 11-P-97553/9-04. Prepared for Health Care Financing Administration. Berkeley, CA: University of California.

NASW (1984). *Standards and guidelines for social work case management for the functionally impaired, professional standards*, Number 12, NASW, Silver Spring, MD.

National Association of Area Agencies (N4A) (1984). *Community-based long-term care statement*. Washington, DC: N4A.

National Association of Area Agencies on Aging (N4A) (1984). *Models of community-based long-term care systems*. Washington, DC: N4A, N.d.

Older Americans Act Amendments of 1984, Section 306, Public Law 98-459.

Palmore, E. (1976). Total chance of institutionalization among the aged. *The Gerontologist, 16*(6): 504–507.

Phillips, B., Baxter, R., & Stephens, S. (1981). *Approach to the client assessment instrument for the national long-term care evaluation.* Princeton, NJ: Mathematica Policy Research.

Price, L.C., & Ripp, H.M. (Nov. 1980). Third year evaluation of the Monroe County Long-Term Care Program, Inc. HCFA Grant No. 05-011-P90—130 and AoA Grant No. 2A-50A. Prepared for Health Care Financing Administration and Administration on Aging. Silver Spring, MD: Macro Systems, Inc.

Region IV Area Agency on Aging (Jan. 1985). Interim evaluation report of case management: Executive summary. St. Joseph, MI.

Rickards, S. (1983). Predicting the client's cost of care: How close do case managers come? Presented at the Annual Meeting of Gerontological Society of America, Nov. San Francisco, CA.

Rivlin, A., Wiener, J. Henley, R., Spence, D. (1988). Caring for the Disabled Elderly: Who Will Pay? Brookings Institution, Washington, D.C.

Sabatino, C. (July 1986). *The black box of home care quality.* Washington, DC: American Bar Association.

Sabatino, C. (1989). Home Care Quality: Putting Public Accountability to the Text, *Generations.* XIII(No 1) pp. 12–16.

Sager, A. (1977). *Estimating the costs of diverting patients from nursing home to home care.* Paper presented at the Annual Meeting of the Gerontological Society, San Francisco, CA.

Schneider, B. (1988). Care planning. *Generations XII*(5): 16–19.

Schneider, B., & Weiss, L. (1982). *The Channeling case management manual.* Prepared for the National Long-Term Care Channeling Demonstration Program, January 18, p. 36.

Schneider, B., Hirsch, C., Richards, S., Sterthous, L.M., Cohen, C., & Wilson, N. (1986). *Beyond assessment: Exploratory Study of Case Management in the Channeling Environment.* Philadelphia: Temple University.

Seidl, F.W., Austin, C.D., & Greene, D.R. (1977). Is home care less expensive? *Health and Social Work,* 2(2): 5–19.

Shealy, M.J., Hicks, B.C., & Quinn, J.L. (Dec. 1979). Triage: Coordinated delivery of services to the elderly, final report. Grant No. H502563. Prepared for National Center for Health Services Research. Plainville, CT: Triage, Inc.

Simpson, D.F. (March 1982). *Case management in long-term care programs.* Washington, DC: Center for the Study of Social Policy.

Simpson, J.B. (1985). State certificate of need programs: Current status. *American Journal of Public Health,* 75(2).

Sklar, B., & Weiss, L.J. (Dec. 1983). *Project Open, Final Report.* San Francisco, CA: Mount Zion Hospital and Medical Center.

Steinberg, R., & Carter, G. (1983). Case management and the elderly. Lexington, MA: Lexington Books, D.C. Heath and Company.

Sterthous, L.M. (1983). *Case management: Variations on a theme.* Philadelphia, PA: Mid-Atlantic Long-Term Care Gerontology Center, Temple University.

Thornton, et al. (1986). *The costs of the National Long-Term Care Demonstration.* Princeton, NJ: Mathematica Policy Research.

U.S. General Accounting Office (Dec. 1982). *The elderly should benefit from expanded home health care but increasing these services will not insure cost reductions*. Pub. No. GAO/IPE-83-1. Washington, DC.

Weissert, W.G. (no date). Estimating the long-term care population: National and prevalence rates and selected characteristics from 1977, 1979 and 1980, and projections to 2000. Working paper of University of North Carolina, School of Public Health in Aging, Chapel Hill, NC.

Weissert, W.G. (1985a). Estimating the long-term care population: Prevalence rates and selected characteristics. *Health Care Financing Review*, 6(4): 83–91.

Weissert, W.G. (Oct. 1985b). Seven reasons why it is so difficult to make community-based long-term care cost-effective. *Health Services Research*, 20(4): 423–433.

Weissert, W.G., & Scanlon, W. (July 1983). *Determinants of institutionalization of the aged*. The Urban Institute Working Paper #1466-21.

Zawadski, R.T., et al. (Dec. 1984). *On Lok Senior Health Services: A community care organization for dependent adults*. A Research and Development Medicare Waiver Demonstration Project Final Report. San Francisco, CA: On Lok.

Zawadski, R.T., & Ansak, M.L. (1984). *On Lok CCODA: A consolidated model*. In Zawadski, R.T. (ed.). *Community-based systems of long-term care*. New York, NY: The Haworth Press.

Index